Dr Alexander Logan

Get Me Into Medical School!

The Medical Schools Guide

© Meddicle Publishing 2015

www.getmeintomedicalschool.com

Cover design by A Logan

Book design by A Logan

Character design by G Young

ISBN-13: 978-0993113819;

ISBN-10: 0993113818

Get Me Into Medical School! Series

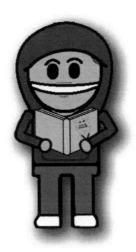

Download the Free App on the App Store

www.getmeintomedicalschool.com

CONTENTS

Introduction

Which medical school should I choose?

After deciding to study medicine your next big decision comes in the form of choosing which medical school, university and consequently city you want to spend the next five to six years of your life living in.
In the United Kingdom you will be permitted a choice of four medical schools to apply to via the UCAS application system and it can be tricky appreciating what differentiates each medical school and knowing where you will be happiest.

The good news is that regardless of where you choose you will (hopefully) qualify with a degree that allows you to practise medicine. The United Kingdom has 34 medical schools each in a different location with slightly different teaching styles, hospitals and facilities. Then there are America, Australia and numerous other English-speaking countries whose medical institutions that you may wish to consider applying to.

Just like using a guide book when visiting a new city this guide book helps you navigate your way through each UK medical school, and some further afield, to help you get a feel for each medical school and city so that you can make a truly informed choice about where to study and ensure that you will be happy and enjoy your time at university.

This book divides each UK medical school into sections covering the medical school itself, the city and the university. Factors such as intercalation, foreign travel and distance of clinical placements, that you may not have considered, are all covered together with details of individual courses and facilities. Each chapter includes opinions from UK medical students studying at the medical school to give a feeling of what life is like in the early and later years.

This guide distils what it is like being a medical student at each UK medical school and provides you with pertinent insight into the positives and negatives of each city, university and medical school before you come to a final decision.

We hope that wherever you choose to study medicine you enjoy both the city and the course.

The Get Me Into Medical School Team
www.getmeintomedicalschool.com

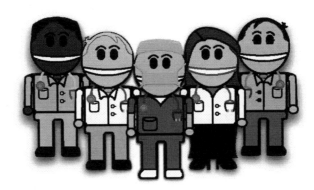

Chapter 1 Choosing a Medical School

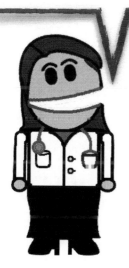

Choosing the medical school that is right for you is a big decision. You will be spending the next five years of your life in the region and may stay longer to work as a doctor. There are many factors that affect your decision, including some you may not have considered. This chapter helps you make the choice that is right for you.

PERSONAL FACTORS

After deciding that medicine is the career for you choosing which medical school is arguably the most important and difficult decision you will face during the application process.

Common motivating factors such as location, peer recommendation and reputation of the medical school will play a pivotal role in your decision making process and it can be difficult to think of other important aspects to consider before making your choice.

In this chapter current medical students and junior doctors have outlined their insider tips and some of the less frequently consider factors that might influence your decision. It is important to remember that every person is different and there is no 'best' medical school, only a medical school that is right for you.

You may already have strong feelings about where you want to go to university. It is worth writing down a shortlist of 8-10 universities then reading this chapter, researching them and whittling the list down to your final selection.

Before looking at the ways in which medical schools differ and their course types let's consider what personal factors you may influence your choice.

Distance From Home Due to the increase in tuition fees and economic climate many people may consider living at home to minimise outgoings on rent, food and prefer the comforts of home. It is important to strike a balance between independence and the proximity of family support and while money might be tight you may miss out on some of the fun of university life by living with your parents (regardless of the improvement in your nutrition and cleanliness).

Location You will be spending at least four years in the city and most graduates choose to undertake their foundation years in the same area that they have studied. It is important that you ensure you can see yourself happily living in the city. You may wish to research local hospitals, areas of the city, entertainment and transport links before making your choice.

Cost of Living Cities such as London can be very expensive for students. The average prices of rent, weekly shops and transport will greatly affect your spending and quality of life. The flip side to this is that these cities tend to be exciting and filled with a wealth of opportunity.

Learning Style This is expanded upon in the following section looking at the course types at each medical school. You may be someone who learns best with self-directed learning or you may prefer to have frequent tutorials. You may prefer to have lectures covering the basic sciences, as seen in traditional courses, or you may want to get straight in to clinical work. Think about which courses best suit your learning style.

Exams Linked to the above point on learning styles it is worth thinking about how useful you consider exams. Some medical schools such as Birmingham have frequent examinations to assess learning while other medical schools offer a more relaxed assessment of students.

Competition You may already be aware of how strong your application is. If you have decided upon medicine at the last minute and don't have as strong an application as your peers you may wish to apply to less competitive medical schools and be tactical with your application. We do not recommend selecting any medical school that you will not be happy to study at.

University Life Do you enjoy large cities or do you prefer smaller, compact locations? Getting lost in a large city or university can be scary and larger year groups may make it harder to meet everyone.

Activities and Interests If you are a keen sports player, athlete, dancer or have another strong interest it is important to research whether the university caters for you. Are there good sports facilities? What is the student union like? Is the nightlife varied and exciting enough for you?

Peer Group Do you want to go to the same university as your close friends or would you prefer to go somewhere by yourself? It is also worth considering what type of students attend the university and whether you will fit in to this tribe. While most universities have students from a wide range of backgrounds older universities such as Oxbridge, Bristol, Edinburgh and Imperial tend to have more middle-class and privately educated students possibly due to the cost of living and their surrounding areas.

Following graduation doctors may undertake the foundation years in any region in the UK. Since students are familiar with the hospitals in their area most choose to stay around the city in which they studied.

MEDICAL SCHOOL FACTORS

There are 34 UK medical schools to choose from. Warwick and Swansea only offer places to postgraduate students leaving 32 medical schools open to both undergraduates and mature students. Durham and St Andrews medical schools only offer preclinical courses with students then moving to one of their partnered medical schools to complete the clinical years.

Some medical schools offer a premedical year for students without science-based A-Levels and some offer a four-year fast-track course known as Graduate-Entry Medicine (GEM) courses for students with a previous degree.

Course type, length and location are common factors considered by students when selecting a medical school. However there are many intricacies and important factors that only reveal themselves when you are at medical school.

Below we discuss the differences between course types and discuss some less common things to consider that have been highlighted by current medical students.

Types of Course

There are three basic types of medical course taught at UK universities: Traditional, Integrated and Problem-Based Learning (PBL). Traditional and Integrated are very similar, with some overlap of their core concepts of lectures and clinical attachments. There are no better or worse course types only personal preference to a style of teaching. It is important to note that learning at university is very different from school and with any method of teaching you will be required to study on your own accord and rely less on didactic teaching as you will have received at school.

Traditional

The first two years (preclinical) are lecture-based covering the basic sciences and anatomy. Limited to establishments such as Oxford, Cambridge and St Andrews, there is a definite preclinical/clinical divide and the preclinical years are taught very rigidly in subjects.

Positives +	Negatives -
• Students get a solid grounding of the theory behind medicine before clinical practice which aids subsequent learning and understanding. • Lectures are sociable and allow students to enjoy university life before visiting academies and taking on clinical responsibilities	• Some students may not enjoy the pure theory • Some scientific detail forgotten by the time students reach clinical years

Integrated

Clinical attachments are integrated with lectures that are focussed on systems of the body. The amount of patient contact increases as the years progress with there still being a slight divide between preclinical and clinical years. This type of course is used by the majority of UK medical schools.

Positives +	Negatives -
• Lectures are focussed and centred around clinical attachments to maximise deep learning. • Early clinical attachments	• Early clinical responsibilities may be too early for some • Same format throughout the course

Problem-Based Learning

Students work through clinical cases in a group rather than learn from didactic lectures. Examples may be linked with clinical attachments. More emphasis is put on self-directed learning and learning from examples. E.g Discuss the management of an 80 year old lady with hypertension.

Universities offering this type of course include Liverpool, Manchester, Glasgow, Queen Mary, Peninsula, Keele, Hull and York, Barts and East Anglia.

Positives +	Negatives -
• Teamwork and self-directed learning is promoted • Relevance to clinical practice	• Dependent on self-directed learning which is a big jump from school teaching • Does not give a solid science-based grounding

Course Length and Degree Awarded

The majority of undergraduate medicine courses are five years in length. Cambridge, Imperial, Oxford, St Andrews and UCL include an extra year of compulsory intercalation and some offer fast-track four year courses for graduates. If you did not undertake science A-Levels some medical schools also offer a premedical or foundation year prior to the standard undergraduate course.

While all medical schools allow you to qualify as a doctor the final degree (and letters that will appear after your name) can differ between each awarding university. For example one may award an MBChB, another may award MBBS and another BM BCh. These all mean the same thing Bachelor of Medicine Bachelor of Surgery (Chirugie) with some recognising the core science component in it's own right. There is absolutely no difference between them, though it can be very confusing when researching and comparing medical schools.

Entry Requirements

Medicine is competitive and universities usually want A grades in science-based subjects. The exact requirements differ between each medical school and it is important that you select a medical school that fits your purpose. Together with grades admission tests are also a major part of securing a place. If you have been struggling with the UKCAT or BMAT you may wish to choose at least one medical school that does not require these as standard to improve your chances of getting a place.

Subtleties other than grades and admission tests include some requiring chemistry and/or biology as mandatory, some accepting A-Level re-sits and some allowing for deferred entry after a gap year. The best way to find out more about a specific medical school is to read the Medical School Guide chapter of this book and to check their respective admission websites.

Other Factors

Graduate Entry The main decision facing graduates is whether to choose a fast-track GEM course or the standard undergraduate course. It is important to note that some medical schools only accept graduate applicants.

Reputation Unlike many jobs that give extra credit to applicants from Oxbridge, Edinburgh, Bristol or London universities your medical degree will be the same whichever university you study at. In practical terms your medical school will have very little effect on your future career other than getting you through medical school and influencing the region that you work in as a graduate.

League Tables The Times and The Guardian Newspapers publish subject-specific university league tables every year. These may be useful for courses such as business, law or languages, where graduates will be facing competitive selection into a wide range of careers, to give students an idea of how a particular university course will affect their career prospects. For medicine, where foundation jobs are closely related to number of medical school graduates and job prospects near 100%, they are virtually irrelevant.

League tables are scored based on average UCAS score for entry, student satisfaction (from the National Student Survey), academic research, staff to student ratio and employability. If you look at the hard figures such as the entry standards or National Student Survey results there is little significant difference between the highest and lowest scoring medical schools. Similarly does the a local international research centre or a high teacher to student ratio make for a better education? The answer is almost certainly no. Interestingly many parents and teachers are influenced by league tables and want students to attend the 'top' medical schools. This is entirely wrong and it is much more important to choose somewhere to study that suits your personal preferences rather than a ranking table.

Academic Research It may be that you are interested in lab-based projects or the research side of medicine. If this is something that you are passionate about it is worth reading the website for the medical school research department and research where the major international research centres are based in the UK. In reality most universities have large research departments that cater for medical students and this shouldn't play a major role in your selection choice.

Local Hospitals As part of your interview practice you will be researching where the local medical school academies are located in the region. Academies are simply a term for the hospitals that take students for their clinical attachments. Some universities send students to hospitals upwards of two hours away from their city of study and these may not be the large teaching hospitals that you are used to seeing. As you may very well be staying in the region to work as a foundation doctor it is vital to have a solid knowledge of the major hospitals and academies in the region. Generally speaking, you should be on the look out for hospitals in pleasant areas which are a commutable distance (30-60minutes) from your home city in case you do not wish to stay in accommodation while on attachment.

Further information on academies can be found in the Career in Medicine Chapter and in the Medical School Guide section of this book and on the medical school course information pages.

Exam Format and Frequency As mentioned in the Personal Factors section medical school examinations vary widely between medical schools. Exams may not be something you have considered when thinking about a medical school but it can greatly affect your enjoyment and time at university. Most medical schools test students using multiple choice SIngle Best Answer or Extended Matching Questions for knowledge and Objective Structured Clinical Examinations (OSCEs) for clinical skills (more on these in the Career in Medicine Chapter). Some medical schools test students frequently such as at the end of each clinical attachment while others rely on you to work hard during the year and only hold major exams at halfway through and at the end of the year.

Year Size Another factor that is often overlooked. Big medical schools sometimes have year sizes nearing four-hundred students and this can make lectures crowded and impersonal. It can also make it difficult to recognise and meet fellow medics and students may get lost in such a large year. Year sizes of around two-hundred allow for socialising and a good atmosphere in lectures and on attachments.

Medicine Abroad One of the highlights of medical school is the medical elective that typically occurs in the penultimate or final year of study. This is an opportunity to go traveling anywhere in the world and experience global healthcare. The timing and length of elective is worth looking up for the medical schools that you are applying to in case there are any restrictions.

Another way to study abroad during medical school is to take part in an Erasmus programme with a European university. This is offered by a select group of UK medical schools and requires a basic understanding of the host language.

Anatomy Teaching Anatomy is one of the cornerstones of medicine and an understanding of the structures in the human body makes learning about diseases and treating patients much easier. It is also a unique experience, enjoyable and particularly important if you think you may wish to be a surgeon. Due to a shortage of donated cadavers and lack of anatomy laboratories at some universities anatomy teaching can vary widely between medical schools. The best teaching is done using cadavers and dissection, guided by anatomy demonstrators and utilising computer aided learning to help understand key-concepts. Poor anatomy teaching is using plastic models and computer software only.

Medical School Facilities New buildings and teaching facilities are usually highlighted on medical school and university websites. It is important that the medical school has a large, accessible medical library, computer facilities and clinical teaching labs that are close to the university campus.

Some medical schools will have invested money in the latest teaching labs, software and facilities. Knowing this may influence your choice and will give you something to talk about at your medical school interview.

UNIVERSITY AND CITY FACTORS

Having considered your personal reasons and information about the medical school a final area you may wish to consider is the university and city of study.

While learning medicine is important it is equally important that you are happy in your chosen location, meet a good set of friends and enjoy your time living and working in your chosen university.

University Type

Just like with types of medical course an important part of choosing a university is to consider how the university is laid out. There are three main types of university: campus, collegiate and city. You will normally only stay in university halls of residence for your first year before moving into rented accommodation in the city. Your first year is lots of fun and you will meet plenty of new people, make sure you enjoy it!

Campus

The university, including accommodation, teaching facilities and leisure facilities, are located in a single site or 'campus' usually outside of the main city.

E.g Nottingham, UEA, Keele and Warwick

Positives +	Negatives -
• Enclosed student community which is safe and fun • Cheap cost of living and plenty of student deals	• Sheltered environment and loads of students can make it distant from the real world • You will need to get used to traveling to hospitals anyway

Collegiate

Students live in independent colleges that provide food, social events and other services. Students are often paired into hospital attachments, lab groups and lectures with fellow college members.

e.g. Cambridge and Oxford

Positives +	Negatives -
• Close community • Colleges provide good support in addition to that provided by the university	• Minimal interaction between colleges and can be cliquey • Traditional college rules may not be to everyone's liking

City

University buildings are located across the city. Typically teaching facilities are in a central university campus and halls of residence are spread across the city.

e.g. Most UK universities

Positives +	Negatives -
• Halls of residence often offer the best parts of collegiate community while allowing mixing of students • You truly integrate with the city	• May require travel to and from lectures • In larger cities it can be overwhelming

Other Factors

Accommodation While most universities are of the city type there is a wide variation in the quality and locality of their halls of residence. Most universities offer a selection of halls ranging from expensive options to cheaper options. Looking through the accommodation pages of your shortlisted medical schools can be fun and exciting as you imagine yourself living there. Your accommodation is important as you need somewhere to relax and socialise and halls of residence or independent housing will be central to this. Make sure you take a tour of the halls if it is offered during an open day and ask current students what their top choices would be. University websites have accommodation pages with photo or video tours that can also help you to make a decision.

Students' Union and Clubs The union usually has its own website listing all the clubs and societies that you may wish to join at the freshers' fair in the first week of term. Some student unions, such as Cardiff and Southampton, have clubs and bars housed within them and are a local haunt for most of the university.

Sports Facilities If you enjoy keeping fit or playing sport you will want to look at the sports facilities offered by each university. Most student gyms will be very busy and it is important that you choose a large enough gym that you are able to attend regularly after paying the subscription. Information on university sports team can be found at www.BUCS.org.uk and if you play sport to a high level it is worth comparing the quality and success of university teams. Fort the more casual sports person most universities have multiple teams of varying levels and medial schools will have their own sports teams that compete in medical school competitions.

Nightlife If you are someone who enjoys going out, hitting the town and socialising larger trendy cities such as Bristol, London, Newcastle, Liverpool or Leeds offer lots of cool bars and night clubs and run plenty of student nights offering drinks deals and fun. If you prefer quiet pubs or bars quieter cities such as Oxford, Cambridge or Warwick may be more to your tastes.

Chapter 2 The Medical Schools Guide

Each of the 34 UK medical schools is slightly different and it is important to find out as much about the course and university as possible before making your final decision. This chapter is best used together with the admissions pages of the medical schools that you are considering.

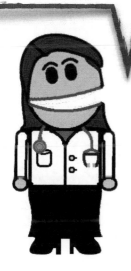

England

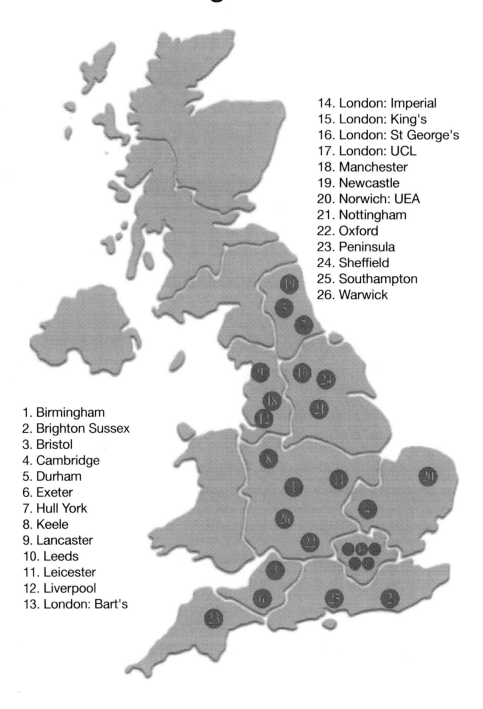

14. London: Imperial
15. London: King's
16. London: St George's
17. London: UCL
18. Manchester
19. Newcastle
20. Norwich: UEA
21. Nottingham
22. Oxford
23. Peninsula
24. Sheffield
25. Southampton
26. Warwick

1. Birmingham
2. Brighton Sussex
3. Bristol
4. Cambridge
5. Durham
6. Exeter
7. Hull York
8. Keele
9. Lancaster
10. Leeds
11. Leicester
12. Liverpool
13. London: Bart's

BIRMINGHAM

UNIVERSITY^{OF} BIRMINGHAM

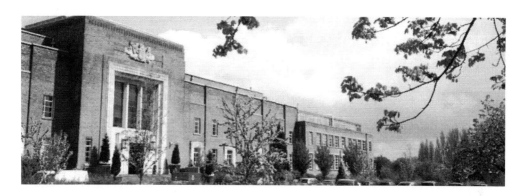

CONTACT DETAILS

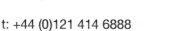

Admissions Tutor
Medical School
The University of Birmingham
Edgbaston
Birmingham B15 2TT

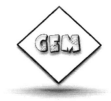

t: +44 (0)121 414 6888
e: medicineadmissions@contacts.bham.ac.uk

http://www.birmingham.ac.uk/students/courses/undergraduate/med/medicine.aspx

Birmingham is in the heart of the midlands and there is plenty to do from shopping at the Bullring to listening to music at Birmingham Symphony Hall. There is a strong emphasis on sports with Aston Villa, Wolves and Birmingham City football clubs, Edgbaston Cricket Ground and Edgbaston Golf Club accessible from the main university campus.

The medical school and surrounding hospitals have seen much recent investment and development. The medical course is integrated and the large military hospitals provide fantastic teaching opportunities.

The university boasts a beautiful campus with modern student accommodation such as Mason's Hall.

Course Information

Course Programmes	Standard (A100) GEM (A101)	**Course Length**	5 years 4 years (GEM)
Course Type	Integrated	**Degree Awarded**	MBChB
Year Size	334	**University Type**	City

Entry Requirements

	Students	Graduates
Typical Offer	A*AA	1st
Required Subjects	Chemistry & Biology	Life science degree
Admission Tests	UKCAT	None

Admission Statistics

	Standard	GEM
Applicants	1500	680
Interviews	1150	100
Places	334	40
Applicants per Place	4:1	17:1
Open Days	July	**International Places** 28

The Interview

	Standard	GEM
Format	MMI	MMI
Length	6 stations, 6 mins (36)	6 stations, 6 mins (36)
When	Nov-March	Nov-March

Course Overview

First and Second Years

The first two years feature modules on the structure and function of the human body. You will learn how each system works and how diseases and medical treatments affect them. Anatomy is taught in small-group sessions using pro-sections.

Ten days each year are spent in the community at GP surgeries, linking theoretical learning to clinical situations with real patients.

Third Year

You will be based in a hospital around Birmingham to further develop your basic clinical skills, history taking and examination skills. You will learn about common diseases and how to diagnose and manage them. Alongside clinical attachments, lectures cover pathology, pharmacology, public health and epidemiology.

Fourth and Fifth Years

You will build on your clinical experiences and rotate through specialities such as Cardiology, Neurology, Psychiatry, Orthopaedics, Oncology, Ear, Nose and Throat and Peri-Operative Care. You will also do further attachments in Obstetrics and Gynaecology, Paediatrics and General Practice. During the final year, you will be able to bring all of your learning and skills together through the Acutely Ill Patient attachment, which is a chance to shadow a foundation doctor, as you prepare to become an F1.

Hospitals

UHB Queen Elizabeth	2 Mins	Alexandra Hospital	25 Mins
Womens' Hospital	2 Mins	Russell's Hall Hospital	25 Mins
Barberry	3 Mins	Sandwell General	25 Mins
UHB Selly Oak	5 Mins	Good Hope Hospital	30 Mins
Royal Orthopaedic Hospital	5 Mins	Walsall Manor Hospital	30 Mins
Birmingham City Hospital	15 Mins	Worcester Acute	30 Mins
Birmingham Children's Hospital	15 Mins	New Cross Wolverhampton	35 Mins
Whittall Street Clinic	15 Mins	Hereford County	75 Mins
Heartland's Hospital	20 Mins	Royal Shrewsbury	75 Mins

Insider's Edge

The medical school is huge and the large year sizes mean that you can feel lost.

The majority of the city's bars, clubs and attractions are centred around Broad Street, a five minute taxi ride from the student area of Edgbaston.

The Bullring is a huge shopping complex accessed through Broad Street and has a whole range of shops. For a slightly more upmarket atmosphere, for those who can afford it, there is the Mailbox just around the corner from Broad Street. The Mailbox is tucked away from busy traffic and offers designer shops, and a number of highly rated hotels and restaurants.

BRIGHTON-SUSSEX

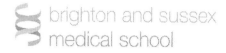

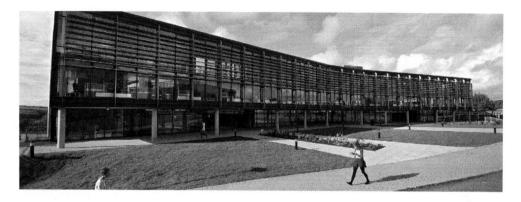

CONTACT DETAILS

BSMS Teaching Building
University of Sussex
Brighton
East Sussex
BN1 9PX

t: +44 (0)1273 643528
e: medadmissions@bsms.ac.uk

http://www.bsms.ac.uk/undergraduate/

Located on the south coast and famed for its pier and pavilion Brighton is a diverse and energetic city with plenty for students to enjoy.

The medical school was established in 2003 and offers a modern, integrated course with a small year size making for a friendly atmosphere.

Students belong to both the universities of Brighton and Sussex and have access to facilities at both. Freshers stay around the Falmer campus which is surrounded by the beautiful South Downs National Park and only a short journey from central Brighton.

Research is important and the medical school has 80 dedicated research staff covering 12 specialities. Key research groups include cancer, primary care and health services, and infection and immunology.

Course Information

Course Programmes	Standard (A100)	Course Length	5 years
Course Type	Integrated	Degree Awarded	BMBS
Year Size	125	University Type	City

Entry Requirements

	Students	Graduates
Typical Offer	AAAb	2:1
Required Subjects	Chemistry & Biology	Life science degree
Admission Tests	BMAT	BMAT

Admission Statistics

	Standard		
Applicants	1400		
Interviews	500		
Places	125	Open Days	June & July
Applicants per Place	11:1	International Places	10

The Interview

Format	Traditional
Length	20 Minutes
When	Jan-March

Course Overview

Phase 1 (Years 1-2)

Phase 1 is based at both the Brighton and Sussex university campuses at Falmer, one of the benefits of being members of two universities in the same city.

The purpose-built teaching facilities at Falmer provide a modern anatomy laboratory, tutorial and seminar rooms, lecture theatres, clinical science laboratories and IT resource suites. Fully equipped consultation rooms, identical to those used in GP surgeries and hospital outpatients departments, provide a setting in which to learn history taking and examination. These are located close to a clinical skills training area, which also houses an advanced patient simulator, computer-controlled to represent normal and abnormal physiology and a realistic response to drugs.

Phase 2 (Years 3-4)

Phase 2 is based at the Education Centre at the Royal Sussex County Hospital in Brighton. During these years, clinical experiences increase and integrated lectures cover sciences and public health.

Phase 3 (Year 5)

Year 5 provides intense clinical and professional preparation for your first year in practice after qualification. Attachments involve joining small clinical teams in medicine, elderly care, surgery, obstetrics, gynaecology, paediatrics, general practice and mental health, where your learning will be based on close involvement with routine clinical cases. Central to your study will be the assessment, diagnosis and treatment of patients presenting to these different areas of practice, acting as a member of the clinical team with the foundation doctors.

Hospitals

Brighton General Hospital	10 Minutes	Eastbourne General Hospital	45 Minutes
Royal Sussex County Hospital	25 Minutes	Redhill Hospital	1 hour
Haywards Heath Princess Royal Hospital	30 Minutes	Chichester Hospital	1 hour
Worthing Hospital	30 Minutes	Hastings Conquest Hospital	1 hour

Insider's Edge

Being small and new, the environment at BSMS is friendly, personal and supportive. Each student has a personal Academic Tutor in years 1 and 2, and a Clinical Academic Tutor for years 3-5. You will really get to know the tutors and hospital doctors and most are more than happy to offer help, guidance and support if needed.

Brighton is a great place to be a student – trying to balance all the nights out and days on the beach or in town with such a challenging course certainly improved my time-management skills! I wouldn't have it any other way though as there's never a dull moment.

The interview consists of:

- A short presentations about BSMS, its curriculum and its admissions process
- A formal 20 minute semi-structured interview
- A student-guided tour of the Falmer campuses (including accommodation)

BRISTOL

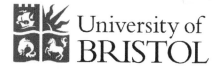

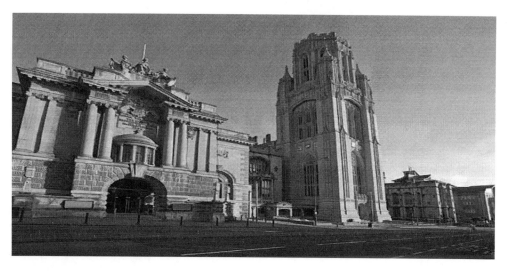

CONTACT DETAILS

Undergraduate Admissions,
Second Floor South,
Senate House,
Tyndall Avenue,
Bristol, BS8 1TH

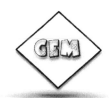

t: +44 (0)117 928 7679
e: med-admissions@bristol.ac.uk

http://www.bristol.ac.uk/medical-school/prospective/

Bristol is famous for Banksy's street art and its stunning architecture such as Clifton Suspension Bridge and the Wills' Memorial Building. Bristol has one of the oldest medical schools in the country and boasts modern facilities and academic excellence with strong hospital teaching and research departments.

Bristol offers modern appeal against a background of rich history and the medical school features an integrated course with focus on lecture-based teaching in the first two years allowing students to learn in a friendly and relaxed setting.

Course Information

Course Programmes	Standard (A100) GEM (A101)	**Course Length**	5 years 4 years (GEM)
Course Type	Integrated	**Degree Awarded**	MBChB
Year Size	232	**University Type**	City

Entry Requirements

	Students	Graduates
Typical Offer	AAAb	2:1
Required Subjects	Chemistry & Biology or Physics	Life science degree
Admission Tests	None	None

Admission Statistics

	Standard	GEM
Applicants	3500	500
Interviews	800	100
Places	232	19
Applicants per Place	15:1	25:1
Open Days	July	**International Places** 19

The Interview

	Students	GEM
Format	MMI	MMI
Length	60 Minutes	60 Minutes
When	Dec-March	Dec-March

Course Overview

Year 1

The first year covers the Human Basis of Medicine (HBoM) and Molecular and Cellular Basis of Medicine. HBoM focusses on communication skills and during this element students visit patients at home and observe GP consultations. Students are mainly based in lectures and labs providing them with the science knowledge base necessary for later teaching. At the end of the fist year students begin to study systems of the body beginning with the cardiovascular system.

Year 2

The second year continues with teaching on systems of the body with week-long hospital placements integrated with lectures. More emphasis is put on clinical skills teaching and around 25% of the curriculum time is set aside for student selected components (SSCs). All students complete one project as a library based research project, the second project is often more practical and chosen from a range of options. Examples are: dissection, deaf studies or applied foreign languages (European).

Years 3-4

Years 3-4 mark a distinct shift in emphasis towards clinically-based teaching, and are intended to provide a firm basis for the development of core clinical skills, including history taking and clinical examination. For the next three years students will spend the majority of their time based at hospitals and in general practice in Bristol and the surrounding areas.

Year 5

Year 5 has been designed to prepare students for their Foundation training and includes the Preparing for Professional Practice (PPP) unit involving a 10 week student assistantship with F1 and F2 doctors and 2 weeks of GP placement. The Elective Period lasts 8 weeks and takes place after finals.

Hospitals

Bristol Royal Infirmary	3 Minutes	Gloucester Royal Hospital	1 Hour
Southmead Hospital	10 Minutes	Cheltenham General	1 Hour
Frenchay Hospital	15 Minutes	Musgrove Park Taunton	1 Hour
Weston Hospital	45 Minutes	Swindon Hospital	1 Hour
RUH Bath	50 Minutes	Yeovil Hospital	1 Hour 15 Minutes

Insider's Edge

Most 1st years live in halls of residence in either Stoke Bishop or Clifton. Stoke Bishop is a good 30-40 minute walk to the medical school across the Downs', whereas Clifton is around a 20 minute walk to the medical school. Student areas of the city include Redland and Clifton where the majority of students rent properties.

Both the halls of residence and student areas feature stunning buildings and are in close proximity to one another making for a strong student community. Wills Hall offers an Oxbridge college feel with its quad and beautiful buildings and rooms.

Bristol is a great place to relax and enjoy yourself whether it is enjoying a beer at the White Lion pub overlooking the Suspension Bridge, jogging around The Downs, attending a drum and bass night at Thekla (a boat converted to a club) or venturing into the surrounding countryside there is something for everyone.

CAMBRIDGE

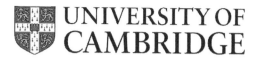

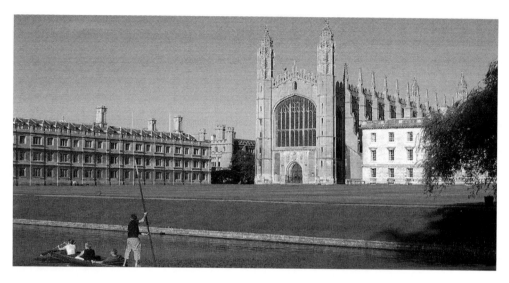

CONTACT DETAILS

University of Cambridge School of Clinical Medicine
Addenbrooke's Hospital, Box 111
Hills Road
Cambridge
CB2 0SP

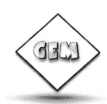

t: +44 (0)122 333 3308
e: admissions@cam.ac.uk

http://www.study.cam.ac.uk/undergraduate/courses/medicine/

The University of Cambridge is recognised as one of the top teaching and research institutions in the world. Students are usually housed in one of the thirty-one colleges for the preclinical years. Cambridge is a fantastic place to study with stunning architecture and plenty to do from punting on the River Cam to visiting a service at King's College Chapel.

The medical course at Cambridge is very traditional, and is separated into Preclinical and Clinical years. The strength of the Cambridge course is that it places great emphasis on the scientific basis behind clinical medicine.

Course Information

Course Programmes	Standard (A100) GEM (A101)	**Course Length**	6 years 4 years (GEM)
Course Type	Traditional	**Degree Awarded**	MB BChir
Year Size	280	**University Type**	Collegiate

Entry Requirements

	Students	Graduates
Typical Offer	A*A*A	2:1
Required Subjects	Chemistry and two of Biology/Human Biology, Physics, Mathematics	Any Degree Subject
Admission Tests	BMAT	BMAT

Admission Statistics

	Standard	GEM
Applicants	2000	250
Interviews	1200	100
Places	280	22
Applicants per Place	6:1	12:1
Open Days	July	**International Places** 22

The Interview

	Students	GEM
Format	Oxbridge	Oxbridge
Length	20 Minutes	20 Minutes
When	Nov-March	Nov-March

Course Overview

At Cambridge, you study the medical sciences first, before learning to apply that knowledge to medical practise as a clinical student.

Years 1-3

The first three years are taught through lectures, practical sessions (including anatomy dissections) and supervisions, with typically 20-25 timetabled teaching hours each week. Supervisions are weekly sessions with a tutor who is an expert in his or her field. Supervision groups usually consist of 2-4 students allowing for personalised feedback and participation.

The emphasis during the clinical years in Cambridge is on learning in a clinical setting: at the bedside, in outpatient clinics and in GP surgeries. Clinical teaching is supported by seminars, tutorials and discussion groups.

Years 4-6

The clinical years (4-6) for students who stay in Cambridge are based at Addenbrooke's Hospital, Cambridge University Hospitals NHS Foundation Trust. As well as being a tertiary hospital with an international reputation for medical excellence, Addenbrooke's is the site of several major biomedical research institutions. You also spend time in other regional NHS hospitals throughout East Anglia, and in general practices in Cambridge and the surrounding region. Roughly half of undergraduates remain in Cambridge while the rest study clinical medicine at hospitals in London or Oxford.

Hospitals

Addenbrooke's Hospital	15 Minutes	Bedford Hospital	55 Minutes
Papworth Hospital	25 Minutes	Luton & Dunstable Hospital	1 Hour 15 Minutes
Hinchingbrooke Hospital	40 Minutes	The Queen Elizabeth Hospital King's Lynn	1 Hour 15 Minutes
West Suffolk Hospital	40 Minutes	Cross University Hospital	1 Hour 15 Minutes
Peterborough District Hospital	55 Minutes	Ipswich Hospital Whipps	1 Hour 30 Minutes

Insider's Edge

Cambridge is a great place to study offering world-leading academic, research, and teaching facilities. The academic focus, while sometimes tiring, can really push you to achieve. The atmosphere, buildings and countless bars within about 5 minutes of the colleges means you feel at home and will get to know all of your year.

Choose your college carefully by going to open days. Colleges differ on many aspects such as accommodation, grants, location and size.

If you are in a smaller college be sure to make friends with medics from the larger colleges so that they can get you tickets for the decadent May balls.

Research your intercalated year carefully to ensure you enjoy this science-based year.

DURHAM

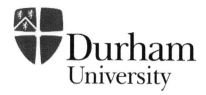

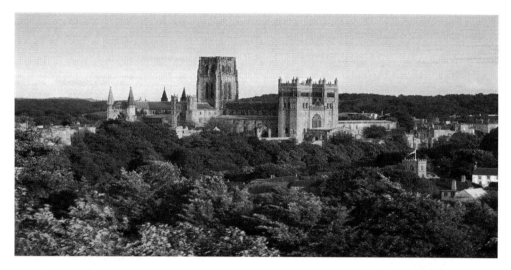

CONTACT DETAILS

Durham University School of Medicine, Pharmacy and Health
Queen's Campus
University Boulevard
Stockton-on-Tees
TS17 6BH

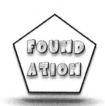

t: +44 (0) 191 33 40353
e: medicine.admissions@durham.ac.uk

https://www.dur.ac.uk/school.health/phase1.medicine/

Durham offers a two-year preclinical course with the clinical years based at Newcastle University.

Medicine at Durham goes back to even before the establishment of the University 175 years ago. The reinstatement of undergraduate medical training in 2001 heralded a new, innovative curriculum in partnership with Newcastle Medical School. Students experience the real world of clinical medicine from the start and the case-led approach emphasises the environment within which the graduating doctor will practice.

Course Information

Course Programmes	Standard (A100) Foundation	**Course Length**	5 years 6 years (Foundation)
Course Type	Integrated	**Degree Awarded**	MBBS
Year Size	100	**University Type**	Collegiate

Entry Requirements

	Students	Graduates
Typical Offer	AAA	2:1
Required Subjects	Chemistry and Biology	Life science degree
Admission Tests	UKCAT	UKCAT

Admission Statistics

	Standard	Foundation
Applicants	500	100
Interviews	250	50
Places	100	10
Applicants per Place	5:1	10:1

Open Days	July	**International Places**	29

The Interview

Format	Traditional
Length	45 Minutes
When	Nov-March

Course Overview

Phase I at Durham is two years long and establishes a core knowledge base for medicine. You will be based in the School of Medicine, Pharmacy and Health at the Queen's Campus, Stockton-on-Tees.

At the end of Phase I you will be integrated with students from Newcastle University and allocated to one of four regional clusters of teaching hospitals (Clinical Base Units) for twelve months of clinical experience as the first part of Phase II.

Phase II is based at Newcastle University and is three years long providing clinical experience in a wide range of NHS hospital and community settings across the region. You will be registered as a Newcastle University student during this period. See Newcastle for further details.

Insider's Edge

The College system encourages people to get involved in societies, sports and socialising. For a small town there is lots to do.

Stockton is a great place to study, although it may seem different to the stereotypical university town. Stockton is small but its compact size allows you to get to know everyone on campus.

EXETER

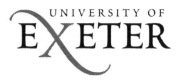

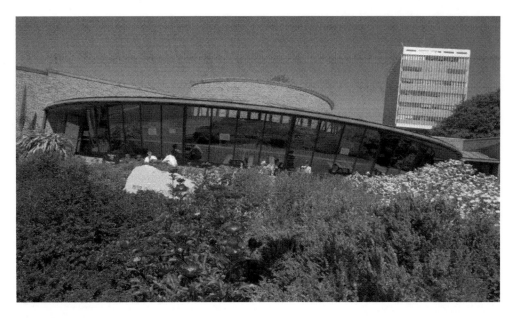

CONTACT DETAILS

Exeter Medical School
University of Exeter Reception
Stocker Road
Exeter EX4 4PY

t: +44 (0) 1392 725500
e: ug-ad@exeter.ac.uk

http://medicine.exeter.ac.uk

Combining the elements from Peninsula Medical School with the University of Exeter, the University of Exeter Medical School welcomed its first entrants in 2013. Students have the opportunity to live and work in locations such as Exeter, Torbay and Truro, experiencing the best of Devon and Cornwall.

The south coast offers a relaxed environment in which to study with beaches and countryside making for fun escapes from University life.

Course Information

Course Programmes	Standard (A100)	Course Length	5 years
Course Type	PBL	Degree Awarded	BMBS
Year Size	130	University Type	City

Entry Requirements

	Students	Graduates
Typical Offer	AAAb	2:1
Required Subjects	Chemistry & Biology or Physics	Life science degree
Admission Tests	UKCAT	GAMSAT

Admission Statistics

	Standard		
Applicants	1800		
Interviews	500		
Places	130	Open Days	April, June, Sept
Applicants per Place	14:1	International Places	10

The Interview

Format	Traditional
Length	20 Minutes
When	Dec & Feb

Course Overview

Years 1 and 2

The first two years give students a solid understanding of clinical medicine. The programme reflects the belief that doctors need to adopt a socially accountable approach to their work and to understand the human and societal impact of disease. Topics are taught using problem-based learning in small groups.

Years 3 and 4

You will rotate through a series of hospital and community placements in the southwest, which provide experiences in a wide range of clinical settings. Learning is patient-centred and small group tutorials and PBL sessions help to consolidate ideas.

Year 5

In your fifth year, you will learn how to be a foundation doctor and start to develop your understanding of principles of practice in the NHS. You'll undertake a series of apprenticeship attachments in hospitals across the southwest to prepare you for after graduation.

Hospitals

Exeter DGH	5 Minutes	Torbay	10 Minutes
Royal Devon and Exeter	5 Minutes	Derriford Hospital	10 Minutes
Truro	10 Minutes		

Insider's Edge

In the first two years, medical students are primarily based at the University's St Luke's Campus in Exeter which is close to the Royal Devon and Exeter Foundation NHS Hospital. Students studying Medical Sciences will also be taught at the Streatham Campus. The two campuses are about a 25-minute walk or a short bus ride apart and buses run frequently.

Students have studied at St Luke's for over 150 years and the campus enjoys a vibrant, atmosphere in which everyone soon gets to know each other. As you walk through the arches of the traditional North Cloisters you will see the lawns of the quadrangle surrounded by modern teaching buildings, including the Medical School buildings.

HULL YORK

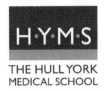

THE HULL YORK
MEDICAL SCHOOL

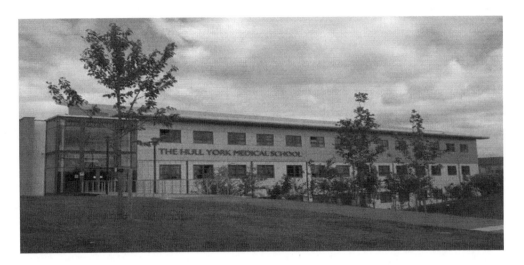

CONTACT DETAILS

John Hughlings Jackson Building
University of York
Heslington
York YO10 5DD

t: +44 (0) 1904 321782
e: admissions@hyms.ac.uk

http://www.hyms.ac.uk

Opened in 2003 Hull York Medical School combines the picturesque city of York and the fast developing, student city of Hull. York is one of the oldest and most beautiful cities in the UK, with its rambling cobbled streets, ancient walls, the famous Minister and pubs. Hull is home to the incredible submarium 'the deep' and a whole area of the city where everything seems aimed at students. Hull and York campuses are around one-hour apart and students are randomly allocated to either campus. The cost of living is low and both rent and living costs can be kept to a minimum.

Course Information

Course Programmes	Standard (A100)	**Course Length**	5 years
Course Type	PBL	**Degree Awarded**	MBBS
Year Size	140	**University Type**	City

Entry Requirements

	Students	Graduates
Typical Offer	AAAb	2:1
Required Subjects	Chemistry & Biology	Life science degree
Admission Tests	UKCAT	UKCAT

Admission Statistics

	Standard		
Applicants	1300		
Interviews	500		
Places	140	**Open Days**	July
Applicants per Place	11:1	**International Places**	10

The Interview

Format	Group task (20mins) then two traditional interviews (10mins each)
Length	40 Minutes
When	Dec - Jan

Course Overview

The five-year course is divided into three phases.

Phase I

In your first two years, you will be based at either the University of Hull or the University of York. Phase I is taught using problem-based learning (PBL). You will be work in groups of eight or nine, alongside an experienced clinical tutor. The PBL sessions are supported by plenaries (lectures), resource sessions and workshops.

Phase II

In years three to four you will gain full exposure to clinical medicine. Hospitals in Hull, York, Grimsby, Scarborough and Scunthorpe allow you to experience a wide range of disease and illness in a diverse social setting. You will work each week in general practice and on the hospital wards.

Phase III

Year five begins with the elective period. When you return from your elective and start your final year at HYMS, you will be the junior member (assistant intern) of a medical team. In this role, you will rotate through general medicine, general surgery and general practice. You will learn how to be a foundation doctor and your working hours will be similar to those of an F1, including on-calls and shift work.

Hospitals

York District Hospital	5 Minutes	Castle Hill Hospital, Hull	15 Minutes
Hull Royal Infirmary	5-10 Minutes	Goole and District Hospital	35 Minutes
Scarborough District General Hospital	10 Minutes		

Insider's Edge

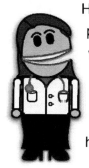 Hull is a lively student city with numerous bars, restaurants, pubs and clubs offering student nights and deals. If that wasn't enough Hull University has an impressive students' union (it has been voted best in the country more than once) with its own nightclub 'Asylum' and bars. From comedy nights to fancy dress balls something is guaranteed to be happening every night of the week.

York is a beautiful city but is more expensive than Hull. There are lots of attractions such as the Viking centre, York dungeons, and the Minster cathedral. There are also many quaint pubs for students to enjoy in York's beautiful surroundings.

The interview consists of three parts: a group task where you are scored on your contribution and two traditional interviews where you are asked common interview questions.

KEELE

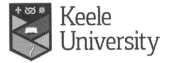
Keele University

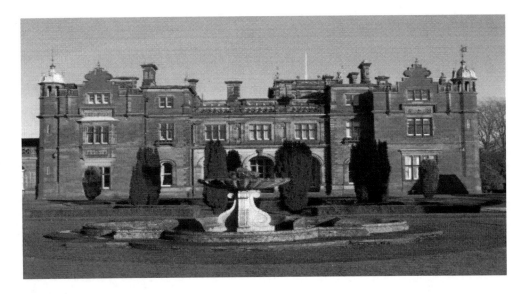

CONTACT DETAILS

School of Medicine
David Weatherall building
Keele University
Staffordshire ST5 5BG

t: +44 (0) 1782 733937
e: medicine@keele.ac.uk

http://www.keele.ac.uk/health/schoolofmedicine/

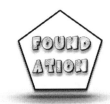

Keele Medical School was established in 2003. Keele is situated in the Midlands between Manchester and Birmingham in the city of Stoke on Trent. Famous for its pottery production, Stoke is a friendly city with a diverse cultural background. Keele is a campus university and regularly wins awards for student popularity with years one and two spent on campus. The three principal buildings are located at the main University campus and at the University Hospital of North Staffordshire (UHNS) campus three miles away.

Course Information

Course Programmes	Standard (A100) Foundation (A104)	**Course Length**	5 years 6 years (Foundation)
Course Type	PBL	**Degree Awarded**	MBChB
Year Size	130	**University Type**	City

Entry Requirements

	Students	Graduates
Typical Offer	AAA	2:1
Required Subjects	Chemistry or Biology & Physics or Maths (or Chem/Bio)	Life science degree
Admission Tests	UKCAT	UKCAT

Admission Statistics

	Standard		
Applicants	2000		
Interviews	500		
Places	130	**Open Days**	June, August, Oct
Applicants per Place	15:1	**International Places**	10

The Interview

Format	MMI
Length	9 stations, 5 mins (55)
When	Dec-March

Course Overview

Medicine is taught using problem-based learning' (PBL) at Keele. Students work in small groups to study clinical situations. Under the guidance of a tutor, students use scenarios to learn relevant topics. Each scenario is the focus for learning for a week, with two or three tutorials devoted to it. From Year 3 onwards PBL develops into case-based learning where the written scenarios are replaced by discussions of patients encountered during clinical placements.

PBL is supported by plenary lectures, seminars, laboratory workshops and a variety of clinical experiences. Placements begin in Year 1 and clinical experiences are built upon throughout the course.

Hospitals

University Hospital of North Staffordshire	7 Minutes	Shrewsbury and Telford Hospitals	50 Minutes
Mid-Staffordshire General Hospitals Foundation Trust	35 Minutes		

Insider's Edge

At Keele University, you start hospital placements in year one. This gives you a chance to see the relevance of your lectures while practising your clinical skills and examining real patients. You also visit GP practices to see how medicine works within the community and gain an insight into local health needs and disease prevention.

Most students in the clinical years live in rented accommodation in Stoke-on-Trent or Shrewsbury. Both these towns are close to Birmingham and Manchester if you want a night out in a larger city.

LANCASTER

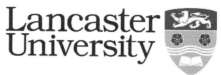

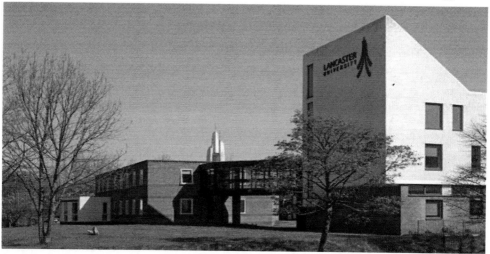

CONTACT DETAILS

Faculty of Health and Medicine
Furness College
Lancaster University
Lancaster
United Kingdom
LA1 4YG

t: +44 (0)1524 593169
e: fhm@lancaster.ac.uk

http://www.lancaster.ac.uk/fhm/

Lancaster medical school is both the smallest and newest UK medical school having been established in 2013 after separating from Liverpool medical school. Lancaster is a vibrant student-friendly city, just ten minutes by bus from the University campus it is filled with pubs, clubs, theatres, markets and shops. Liverpool, Manchester and the Lake District are easily accessible for larger city life or weekend retreats.

Course Information

Course Programmes	Standard (A100)	**Course Length**	5 years
Course Type	PBL	**Degree Awarded**	MBChB
Year Size	50	**University Type**	Campus

Entry Requirements

	Students	Graduates
Typical Offer	AAAb	2:1
Required Subjects	Chemistry and Biology	Life science degree
Admission Tests	BMAT	BMAT

Admission Statistics

	Standard		
Applicants	500		
Interviews	200		
Places	50	**Open Days**	Feb-July
Applicants per Place	10:1	**International Places**	4

The Interview

Format	MMI
Length	12 stations, 5 mins (60) Plus 20 minute group task
When	Dec-March

Course Overview

Medicine is taught using problem-based learning' (PBL) at Lancaster.

Year 1 The Foundations of Medicine

In Year 1, students are based primarily at the University. Through eleven 2-week PBL modules, they are introduced to key concepts in biomedical and social science, and learn about normal structure and function of the human body.

Years 2-4 Learning to Diagnose and Manage Illness

In year 2, students are on campus Monday and Friday, spend two days per week on hospital placement and spend one day per week on Community-related activities, including several days in GP placements, community clinical teaching (CCT) sessions and two community-related assessments. Year 3 comprises five rotations, each of which includes clinical teaching, related PBL and supporting tutorials and lectures: Women and Children, Care of the Elderly, Managing long-term conditions (a GP placement), Therapeutics and Sexual Health, Community Mental Health. In Year 4, students spend a minimum of three days a week in hospital and one day a week in General Practice. Finals are sat at the end of Year 4 followed by a 5-week elective period.

Year 5 Apprenticeship-Style, Intensive Clinical Experience

In Year 5, students undertake five clinical attachments, two of which are Selectives in Advanced Medical Practice (SAMPs).

Students can choose to follow SAMPs in a wide variety of different clinical specialities, providing them with the opportunity to explore different potential medical careers during the course of their undergraduate degree.

Each attachment consists of 7 weeks of intensive clinical experience. A portfolio is used to guide and assess student learning. Students take responsibility for their own learning, engaging in reflective practice, to prepare them for life-long learning.

Hospitals

Lancaster Royal Infirmary	2 Minutes
Furness General Hospital	35 Minutes

Insider's Edge

At Lancaster the small year group of 50 people makes learning easier and more personal; it has allows you to get to know all of your peers and staff within the medical school and the medical school offers a very good support network for learning. The teaching you receive at Lancaster is excellent, and the way the curriculum is designed means your interest is kept up for the duration of the course because of the early mix of clinical and academic work via PBL.

LEEDS

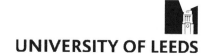

UNIVERSITY OF LEEDS

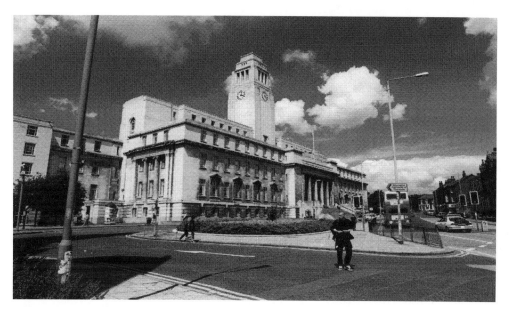

CONTACT DETAILS

The Admissions Section
School of Medicine
Room 7.09, Level 7
Worsley Building, University of Leeds, Leeds, LS2 9JT

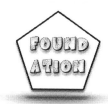

t: +44 (0)113 343 4379
e: ugmadmissions@leeds.ac.uk

http://www.leeds.ac.uk/medicine/index.html

Leeds is a young and vibrant city housing a huge student population. Medicine at Leeds benefits from the large Leeds General Infirmary and surrounding hospitals and the integrated course offers students a solid grounding in medicine.

There is plenty to do with countless clubs and bars for nightlife and the surrounding Yorkshire Dales providing a quick retreat from city life. Leeds offers a Foundation year partnered with Bradford University for students without science-based A-Levels.

Course Information

Course Programmes	Standard (A100) Foundation (at Bradford)	**Course Length**	5 years 6 years (Foundation)
Course Type	Integrated	**Degree Awarded**	MBChB
Year Size	220	**University Type**	City

Entry Requirements

	Students	Graduates
Typical Offer	AAA	2:1
Required Subjects	Chemistry	Life science degree
Admission Tests	UKCAT	UKCAT

Admission Statistics

	Standard		
Applicants	3800		
Interviews	500		
Places	220	**Open Days**	June & October
Applicants per Place	17:1	**International Places**	20

The Interview

Format	MMI
Length	8 stations, 7 mins (60)
When	Dec-Feb

Course Overview

Years 1-2

Year one includes the study of body systems and integrates anatomy dissection with radiology, physiology, clinical assessment and pharmacology.

During year two your understanding of clinical medicine will be developed. Exposure to clinical practice will help to develop history taking, examination and practical skills.

Years 3-4

In year three you will integrate clinical skills and knowledge by undertaking five junior clinical placements, each lasting five weeks. Placements include Integrated Medicine, Surgery and Perioperative Care, Elderly and Rehabilitation Care, Primary Care and Special Senses.

RESS (Research Evaluation and Special Studies) is a core curriculum research strand which spans all five years of the programme. Students undertake an 18-month project in year four which continues through to year five. The projects aim to improve the quality of healthcare in any part of the service related to the clinical specialties studies. Projects may be linked to year four electives, to include an international healthcare aspect with time spent abroad, or take shape as a research study, clinical audit or a public health project.

Year Five

Year five involves three eight-week clinical placements where you work as an 'assistant' making the transition from student to a qualified practitioner. These longer placements help to build strong relationships with clinical teams.

Hospitals

Leeds General Infirmary	On campus	Pinderfields Hospital	30 Minutes
St James' University Hospital	10 Minutes	Huddersfield Royal Infirmary	30 Minutes
Dewsbury and District Hospital	30 Minutes	Bradford Royal Infirmary	35 Minutes
Pontefract Hospital	30 Minutes	Harrogate Hospital	35 Minutes
Calderdale Royal Hospital	30 Minutes	Airedale Hospital	55 Minutes

Insider's Edge

Leeds medical school provides a comprehensive, well-structured and challenging course integrating patient contact at an early stage. Even in the preclinical years teaching is very clinically orientated through a systems based curriculum which uses a variety of teaching methods combined with an element of self directed learning to provide a stimulating course. The clinical years consists of dedicated small group teachings thus giving you the opportunity to develop yourself professionally to become a competent foundation doctor.

If you are into your rugby or football, Leeds is the place for you, with Football at Elland Road and Leeds' Rhino's to support. Headingley boasts Premiership rugby league and union, as well as test match and ODI cricket. For those interested in the arts, there are two large theatres which so a plethora of various stage productions including the much acclaimed Opera North.

LEICESTER

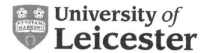

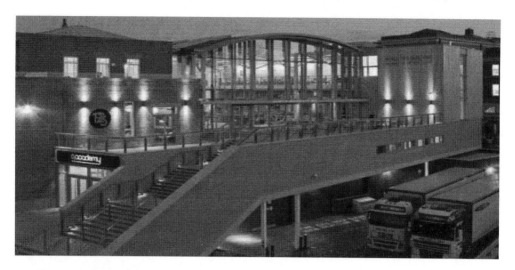

CONTACT DETAILS

University of Leicester Medical School
Maurice Shock Building
PO Box 138
University Road
Leicester
LE1 9HN

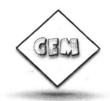

t: +44 (0)116 252 2969
e: med-admis@le.ac.uk

http://www2.le.ac.uk/departments/msce/undergraduate/medicine

Leicester is a lively, culturally diverse city with a huge range of pubs, clubs, restaurants, cinemas and theatres. The opening of the striking Curve Theatre, and the regeneration of the city's cultural quarter, can be seen alongside the established museums and galleries in the city.

Students tend to live in the leafy suburb of Oadby located a short distance from the main university campus. The medical school benefits from three large teaching hospitals located in the city itself.

Course Information

Course Programmes	Standard (A100) GEM (A101)	Course Length	5 years 4 years (GEM)
Course Type	Integrated	Degree Awarded	MBChB
Year Size	180	University Type	City

Entry Requirements

	Students	Graduates
Typical Offer	AAAb	2:1
Required Subjects	Biology & Chemistry	Any degree subject
Admission Tests	UKCAT	UKCAT

Admission Statistics

	Standard	GEM
Applicants	2000	500
Interviews	750	120
Places	180	64
Applicants per Place	11:1	8:1
Open Days	July & Sept	International Places 28

The Interview

	Students	GEM
Format	MMI	MMI
Length	8 stations, 7 mins (60)	8 stations, 7 mins (60)
When	Dec-Feb	Dec-Feb

Course Overview

In 2015/16 the undergraduate course at Leicester underwent a significant reform in how medical teaching was delivered. This was done to reflect the publication of the Francis Report and aims to produce doctors who are caring and possess social responsibility.

Phase 1

Phase 1 is modular, over five semesters for the five-year course and three semesters for the four-year course. In the five-year course there are 26 core modules, and several Student Selected Components. The four-year course has only 20 core modules and one Special Study Module, in recognition of graduates' prior learning.

Phase 2

You will spend nearly all of your time in Phase 2 in long clinical attachments in hospitals and the community that maximise your chances to learn. In the community you will work as part of the primary care team. In hospitals you will be attached to a series of 'Teaching Partnerships'. These are groups of two or three clinicians from different specialties, whose clinical background will provide a wide range of experiences. You will collate a 'portfolio' of written patient studies as you go along.

Hospitals

Leicester Royal Infirmary	5 Minutes	Pilgrim Hospital, Boston	1 hour 45 Minutes
Glenfield Hospital	15 Minutes	Lincoln Hospital	1 hour 30 Minutes
Leicester General Hospital	10 Minutes	Peterborough Hospital	1 hour 5 Minutes
Kettering General Hospital	45 Minutes	Burton Hospital	1 hour
Northampton General Hospital	1 hour	Bedford Hospital	1 hour 30 Minutes

Insider's Edge

The medical student society is very active and runs regular social events including the famous 'pyjama pub crawl'.

Do all the form filling before you arrive at Leicester such as ID badges, society forms and health forms to save you time and help you adjust better when you arrive.

Research accommodation halls and attend open days to get a feel for the city and University so that you make an informed choice about studying at Leicester.

LIVERPOOL

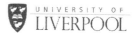

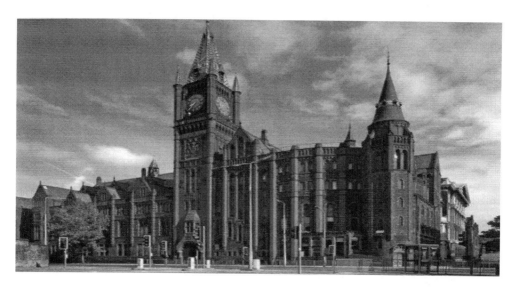

CONTACT DETAILS

School of Medicine
MBChB Office
Cedar House
Ashton Street
Liverpool L69 3GE

t: +44 (0)151 795 4370
e: mbchb@liv.ac.uk

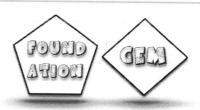

http://www.liv.ac.uk/medicine/undergraduate/

The home of The Beatles, Liverpool is an exciting city with two cathedrals and two of Europe's most successful football teams. The Liverpool ONE complex dominates the city centre and includes designer shops, bars, restaurants and a cinema complex.

The university has benefitted from considerable investment, boasting modern library and sports facilities. The medical school has seen investment in its facilities with new lecture theatres, computer centres, the state-of-the-art Human Anatomy Resource Centre (HARC) and the Centre for Excellence in Developing Professionalism (CEDP).

Course Information

Course Programmes	Standard (A100) Foundation GEM (A101)	**Course Length**	5 years 6 years (Foundation) 4 years (GEM)
Course Type	PBL	**Degree Awarded**	MBChB
Year Size	300	**University Type**	City

Entry Requirements

	Students	Graduates
Typical Offer	AAAb	2:1
Required Subjects	Chemistry and Biology	Life science degree
Admission Tests	None	GAMSAT

Admission Statistics

	Standard	GEM
Applicants	2500	500
Interviews	1200	100
Places	300	40
Applicants per Place	8:1	12:1
Open Days	July	**International Places** 24

The Interview

	Students	GEM
Format	Traditional	Traditional
Length	20 minutes	20 minutes
When	Nov-Feb	Nov-Feb

Course Information

Phase One

Year one introduces you to the science and practice of medicine through a series of PBL clinical cases. You will learn about sciences such as biochemistry, physiology and anatomy. Weekly classes in a specially designed clinical skills centre introduce you to basic clinical methods.

Phase Two

Years two, three and four progress through four stages. Firstly, you understand how healthy bodies normally develop and function. Secondly, you learn to recognise health problems. Thirdly, you develop the skills needed to diagnose illness and disease. Finally, you learn to manage patients. Hospital and community-based clinical experience support your learning and give you plenty of opportunities to interact with real patients.

Phase Five

Year Five is your final year in which you prepare to practise medicine through intensive clinical experience in hospitals and the community.

Hospitals

Royal Liverpool University Hospital	<5 Minutes	Whiston Hospital	40 Minutes
Liverpool Women's Hospital	10 Minutes	Warrington Hospital	50 Minutes
Arrowe Park Hospital	25 Minutes	Southport Hospital	50 Minutes
Alder Hey Children's Hospital	25 Minutes	Countess of Chester Hospital	1hr
Aintree University Hospital	30 Minutes	Blackpool Hospital	1hr 30 Minutes

Insider's Edge

At Liverpool you study by problem-based learning. You'll work in small groups of about 10 with a facilitator, who is usually a doctor. You have a scenario which you 'mind map' together and then set your own learning objectives, go off and research your objectives from books or the internet and a week later you come back and present your findings.

There is loads to do in Liverpool and the nightlife is incredible. The people are all really friendly. Chester and The Wirral offer lots of good day trips and Liverpool has great transport links with an accessible airport and a two-hour train to London.

LONDON: BARTS

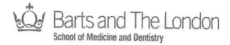

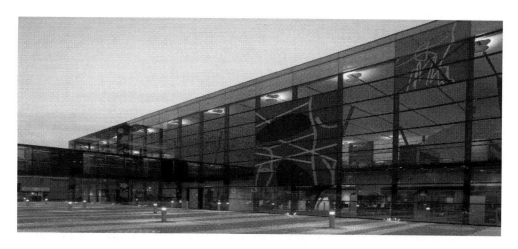

CONTACT DETAILS

Barts and The London School of Medicine & Dentistry
Garrod Building, Turner Street, Whitechapel
London
E1 2AD

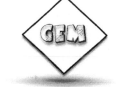

t: +44 (0)20 7882 8478
e: smdadmissions@qmul.ac.uk

http://www.smd.qmul.ac.uk

Barts and The London School of Medicine and Dentistry brings together St Bartholomew's Hospital, which dates back to 1123, and The London Hospital Medical College, founded in 1785, the oldest medical school in England and Wales.

The two hospitals lie in the City and the East End respectively, meaning students are exposed to a wide diversity of people and their problems.

Barts and The London is part of Queen Mary, the only university in London to offer extensive campus-based facilities. This promotes a sense of community and encourages an active social life.

Course Information

Course Programmes	Standard (A100) GEM (A101)	**Course Length**	5 years 4 years (GEM)
Course Type	Integrated	**Degree Awarded**	MBBS
Year Size	253	**University Type**	Campus

Entry Requirements

	Students	Graduates
Typical Offer	AAAb	2:1
Required Subjects	Chemistry or Biology	Life science degree
Admission Tests	UKCAT	UKCAT

Admission Statistics

	Standard	GEM
Applicants	2500	1500
Interviews	800	200
Places	253	40
Applicants per Place	10:1	30:1
Open Days	July	**International Places** 23

The Interview

	Students	GEM
Format	Traditional	Selection Centre (Shared with Warwick)
Length	15 minutes	Half-Day
When	Jan-Feb	Feb

Course Overview

Phase 1 (Years 1-2)

Phase 1 is taught using a series of systems-based modules which introduce the basic biological sciences. Students regularly attend GP practices where they gain early clinical exposure.

Phase 2 (Years 2-4)

You will attend one of the teaching hospitals to gain further exposure to clinical medicine. Your clinical skills will benefit from working alongside clinical teams both in the hospital and also within community placements.

Phase 3 (Year 5)

The final year of the programme provides students with clinical and community placements, practical skills and first hand experience of the working life of a first year Foundation Year (FY1) doctor. Students are placed in the hospital and firm where they will be based for their FY1 training. During this time, they shadow the current FY1 Doctor.

Following finals you will complete a four-week elective and this is followed by a further four-week hospital placement shadowing the FYI doctor they will be replacing following graduation.

Hospitals

Barts and The London Hospitals	10 Minutes	King George, Essex	60 Minutes
Newham University Hospital	35 Minutes	Colchester Hospital, Essex	85 Minutes
Homerton University Hospital	40 Minutes	The Princess Alexandra Hospital, Essex	90 Minutes

Insider's Edge

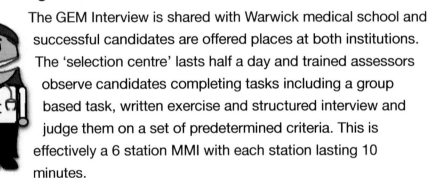 The GEM Interview is shared with Warwick medical school and successful candidates are offered places at both institutions. The 'selection centre' lasts half a day and trained assessors observe candidates completing tasks including a group based task, written exercise and structured interview and judge them on a set of predetermined criteria. This is effectively a 6 station MMI with each station lasting 10 minutes.

Freshers gain the city experience but the fun of campus life with the majority of first years staying at the Mile End campus.

Bart's has a large clinical and communication's skills suite which is available to book throughout the year, these get very busy near exams, the staff are very accommodating and keen to help.

There is a big medical library on the Whitechapel campus with lots of computers. The library at Bart's is smaller but is generally more preferred by students as it is the original medical school library on the Bart's site (with Oak panelling). There is also a big library at the Mile End campus of Queen Mary University which is available to medical students.

LONDON: IMPERIAL

Imperial College
London

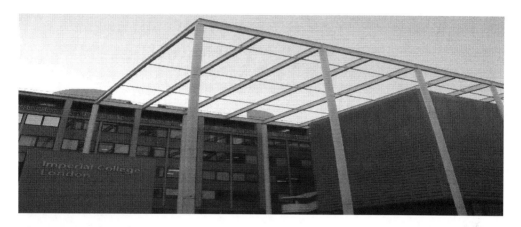

CONTACT DETAILS

Imperial College London,
School of Medicine,
South Kensington Campus,
London SW7 2AZ

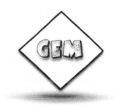

t: +44 (0)20 7594 7259
e: medicine.ug.admissions@imperial.ac.uk

http://www1.imperial.ac.uk/medicine/teaching/undergraduate/

Situated in the capital Imperial College School of Medicine was formed by merging Imperial College with the medical schools of St Mary's and Charing Cross. The standard undergraduate course lasts six years and includes a compulsory intercalated BSc.

The university campus holds state-of-the-art facilities and amenities including a multi-storey gym and refurbished halls of residence next to Hyde Park and the Royal Albert Hall. The medical school has it's own union in addition to the students' union in addition to all that London has to offer.

Course Information

Course Programmes	Standard (A100) GEM (A101)	**Course Length**	6 years 4 years (GEM)
Course Type	Integrated	**Degree Awarded**	MBBS (BSc)
Year Size	277	**University Type**	Campus

Entry Requirements

	Students	Graduates
Typical Offer	AAAb	2:1
Required Subjects	Chemistry or Biology	Life science degree
Admission Tests	BMAT	UKCAT

Admission Statistics

	Standard	GEM
Applicants	2000	1000
Interviews	650	120
Places	277	45
Applicants per Place	7:1	22:1
Open Days	Feb, Apr & July	**International Places** 21

The Interview

	Students	GEM
Format	Traditional	Traditional
Length	15 minutes	15 minutes
When	Jan-Apr	Nov-Jan

Course Overview

Years 1 - 2

During the first year you will begin an integrated programme consisting of themes covering the three main elements of the core course: Scientific Basis of Medicine; Doctor and Patient; and Clinical Experience.

In the second year you progress to your first hospital-based clinical attachment where you begin to apply your knowledge and skills.

Year 3

This year consists of three 10-week clinical attachments, which may be at any of the hospitals opposite.

You also continue to study systems and topics with a programme of live lectures and interactive online learning delivered alongside the clinical attachments.

Year 4 (BSc Degree)

You will spend this year working towards the BSc undertaking a series of modules and a supervised research project or specialist course in an area of particular scientific or medical interest.

Year 5

There is a dedicated pathology course at the start of the fifth year covering essential clinical pathology followed by 10 clinical specialties.

Year 6

The final year consists of seven three-week clinical attachments and the eight-week elective period which may be spent in the UK or overseas.

Hospitals

Royal Brompton	5 Minutes	Hammersmith	13 Minutes
Chelsea & West Minster	6 Minutes	Central Middlesex	17 Minutes
St Mary's	7 Minutes	Ealing	23 Minutes
Charing Cross	8 Minutes	Hillingdon	28 Minutes
St Charles	11 Minutes	St Peter's & Ashford	36 Minutes
West Middlesex	12 Minutes	Northwick Park & St. Mark's	36 Minutes

Insider's Edge

Beit Hall is one of the most sociable Halls to live in. The Union bar is located next door and the beautiful quad offers a great place to sit out on the grass with friends on a warm summer's day. Medical lecture theatres are also only a five minute walk.

Make sure you apply for your Freshers Fortnight Passport early and attend as many events as possible. You will enjoy meeting and mingling with your classmates and with people from across the years.

LONDON: KING'S COLLEGE

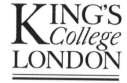

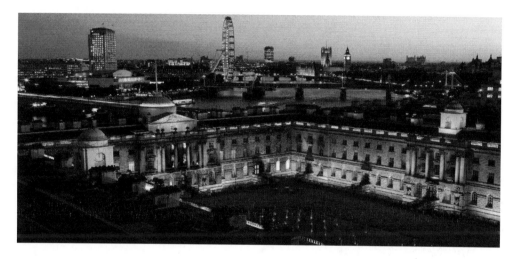

CONTACT DETAILS

King's College London School of Medicine

Stamford St,

London SE1 8WA

t: +44 (0)207 848 7000
e: prospective@kcl.ac.uk
http://www.kcl.ac.uk/medicine/index.aspx

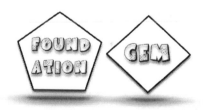

King's College London was founded in 1829 and is the largest centre for the education of doctors, dentists and other healthcare professionals in Europe. It was formed by an amalgamation of Guy's, King's and St Thomas' Hospitals.

Today the School of Medicine has a faculty of 550 academic staff organised within 12 research and teaching divisions which have internationally renowned research programmes.

The hospital has one of the busiest Accident and Emergency Departments in London and since 2012 has been the subject of the reality Channel 4 documentary '24 Hours in A&E'.

Course Information

Course Programmes	Standard (A100) Foundation (A101) GEM (A102)	**Course Length**	5 years 6 years (Foundation) 4 years (GEM)
Course Type	Integrated	**Degree Awarded**	MBBS
Year Size	335	**University Type**	City

Entry Requirements

	Students	Graduates
Typical Offer	AAAb	2:1
Required Subjects	Chemistry & Biology	Any degree subject
Admission Tests	UKCAT	UKCAT

Admission Statistics

	Standard	GEM
Applicants	4500	850
Interviews	1000	100
Places	345	28
Applicants per Place	13:1	9:1
Open Days	July	**International Places** 29

The Interview

	Students	GEM
Format	MMI	MMI
Length	10 stations 6 minutes (60)	10 stations 6 minutes (60)
When	Jan-March	Jan-March

Course Overview

The course is divided into 5 phases over 5 years. For GEM students the first two years are compressed.

Phase 1

Over the first year you will be introduced to the cardiovascular, respiratory, muscular, skeletal, gastrointestinal, renal and nervous systems; immunology and pathology and practice of medicine including psychology, sociology, statistics and ethics.

Phase 2

Over three terms, basic science is studied in a clinical context. You will be presented with a new clinical scenario every week. The clinical scenarios are grouped into systems areas and cover cardiovascular and respiratory medicine, gastrointestinal and renal medicine, metabolism and nutrition.

Phase 3

Phase 3 begins with an introductory course in clinical skills. You will then undertake three 10 or 12-week clinical rotations focussing on different aspects of clinical medicine.

Phase 4

Phase 4 consists of three 13-week rotations in child health, development and ageing; emergency medicine, trauma and locomotion; and reproductive and sexual health.

Phase 5

The year begins with an eight-week elective placement which may be taken in any specialty you choose, almost anywhere in the world. On your return, you undertake three eight-week Student Assistantships in Medicine, Surgery, and General Practice.

Hospitals

Guy's Hospital	2 Minutes	King's College Hospital	20 Minutes
St Thomas' Hospital	10 Minutes	Canterbury	90 minutes

Insider's Edge

The main hub of the medical school is located at the Guy's campus near London Bridge. Most students live around the university campus in halls at Wolfson House and Great Dover Street (10mins from the main campus).

Students can relax on campus at Guy's Bar, in 'The Spit' and can go to Borough Market for lunch after lectures on Fridays.

The virtual campus e-learning resource is extremely useful keeping you up to date and makes it easy to stay on top of the workload.

LONDON: ST GEORGE'S

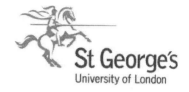

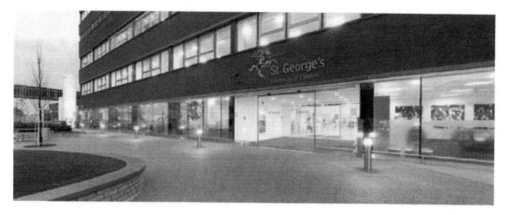

CONTACT DETAILS

St George's University of London,

Cranmer Terrace,

London SW17 0RE

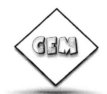

t: +44 (0)20 8725 2333

e: enquiries@sgul.ac.uk

http://www.sgul.ac.uk/courses/undergraduate

In 1733 St. George's Hospital opened in Lanesborough House at Hyde Park Corner and has been training medical students ever since.

Now located in the suburb of Tooting, SGUL has all the excitement that London has to offer, with a friendly student atmosphere. The medical school offers a balanced course with particular emphasis on clinical and communication skills early on.

The medical school is relatively small making for a friendly atmosphere and focus is firmly placed on medical training with nurses, paramedics, physiotherapists and pharmacists training at the same campus.

Course Information

Course Programmes	Standard (A100) GEM (A101)	**Course Length**	5 years 4 years (GEM)
Course Type	Integrated	**Degree Awarded**	MBBS
Year Size	135	**University Type**	City

Entry Requirements

	Students	Graduates
Typical Offer	AAAb	2:1
Required Subjects	Chemistry or Biology	Any degree subject
Admission Tests	UKCAT	GAMSAT

Admission Statistics

	Standard	GEM
Applicants	1400	900
Interviews	800	350
Places	135	90
Applicants per Place	10:1	10:1
Open Days	July	**International Places** 29

The Interview

	Students	GEM
Format	MMI	MMI
Length	8 stations, 5 mins (40)	8 stations, 5 mins (40)
When	Dec-April	Dec-April

Course Overview

The course is underpinned by four main themes: Basic and Clinical Sciences, Patient and Doctor, Community and Population Health and Personal and Professional Development.

Years 1 - 2

In years one and two, the emphasis is on lectures, tutorials and group activity with short clinical and community-based placements.

Year 3

From year three the emphasis shifts towards a combination of problem based learning and student selected components, mixed with clinical attachments. Students have the opportunity in their fourth year to undertake an intercalated BSc of their choice.

Years 4-5

In years four and five the focus is on clinical attachments, again with complementary lectures running in parallel.

During the final year all students undertake an elective. This is an opportunity for you to explore an aspect of medicine of particular interest to you, anywhere in the world.

Hospitals

St. George's Hospital	2 Minutes	Tolworth Hospital	20 Minutes
Springfield University Hospital	5 Minutes	St. Peter's Hospital Chertsey	25 Minutes
St. Helier Hospital	10 Minutes	Redhill and Crawley Hospitals	30 Minutes
Kingston Hospital	15 Minutes	Frimley Park Hospital	40 Minutes
Mayday Hospital, Croydon	20 Minutes		

Insider's Edge

Rent is affordable around the main campus and it is easy to find a large house to share with three or four students. Often, student houses get passed down from year to year to new students and many St George's students live in the area so it is easy to meet up in one of the local pubs after class.

With central London on the doorstep, there is always something exciting to do while students avoid the high costs of living in the centre.

LONDON: UCL

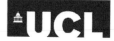

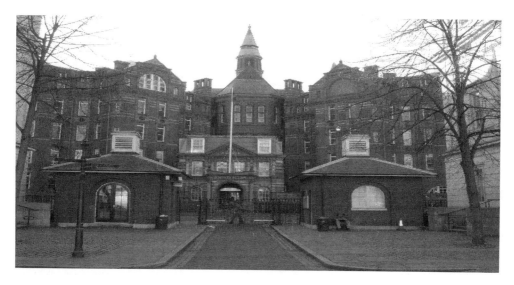

CONTACT DETAILS

Medical Admissions Office
Medical School University College London
Gower Street
London
WC1E 6BT

t: +44 (0)20 7679 0841
e: medicaladmissions@ucl.ac.uk
http://www.ucl.ac.uk/medicalschool/

University College London Medical School was formed from Middlesex Hospital, University College Hospital and the Royal Free Hospital. These institutions combine a rich history of science and medicine with advanced clinical practice. UCL medical school has been producing medical students since 1828 and was one of the first to admit women on equal terms with men.

The medical school is split across three campuses around the teaching hospitals of the Royal Free in Hampstead, the Whittington in Archway and University College Hospital in Bloomsbury.

Course Information

Course Programmes	Standard (A100)	**Course Length**	6 years
Course Type	Integrated	**Degree Awarded**	MBBS BSc
Year Size	322	**University Type**	City

Entry Requirements

	Students	Graduates
Typical Offer	A*AAb	2:1
Required Subjects	Chemistry and Biology	Any subject
Admission Tests	BMAT	BMAT

Admission Statistics

	Standard		
Applicants	2400		
Interviews	700		
Places	322	**Open Days**	June
Applicants per Place	8:1	**International Places**	29

The Interview

Format	Traditional
Length	15 minutes
When	Dec-March

Course Overview

Years 1 - 2

Years one and two are known as 'Fundamentals of Clinical Science' and you will learn about basic clinical sciences. There are opportunities for early patient contact from year one.

Year 3

The medical school offers a range of one year intercalated BSc programmes. UCL medical students (except those who are already UK graduates) are required to take an intercalated BSc as a compulsory part of their six year MBBS programme after completion of Year two.

Year 4

This year aims to integrate knowledge of the clinical sciences into clinical practice and, features clinical attachments and integrated lectures.

Year 5

The theme of year five is 'the life cycle'. A large part of the year is dedicated to beginnings of life, through women's health and child health, but a substantial amount of time is also spent learning about family health, the brain and behaviour.

Year 6

The final year is designed to ensure you have opportunities to think and act like a doctor and to practise and reflect on the areas that will be of use to you on becoming an FY1 doctor.

Hospitals

University College Hospital	5 Minutes	Whittington Hospital	30 Minutes
Royal Free Hospital	30 Minutes		

Insider's Edge

There are many halls of residence in central London that are walking distance from the medical school and some in Camden, a short bus or tube ride away. They are of a good standard and are competitively priced. After the first year most students live in privately rented flats in central or north London. Many graduates do not live in halls in the first year and do not find that this hinders the social aspect of the course.

The main UCL students' union has bars and restaurants that medical students use. In addition there are medical school bars on Huntley Street and at the Royal Free Hospital. For those who enjoy history Jeremy Bentham's embalmed body is on display in the main UCL quad building.

MANCHESTER

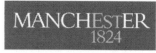

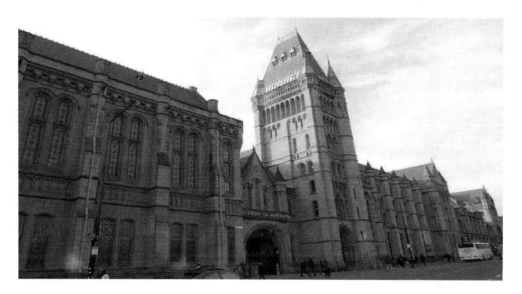

CONTACT DETAILS

Manchester Medical School
The University of Manchester
Stopford Building
Oxford Road
Manchester
M13 9PT

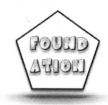

t: +44 (0)161 275 5025
e: ug.medicine@manchester.ac.uk

http://www.mms.manchester.ac.uk/undergraduate/

Manchester medical school offers a modern, problem-based learning course in a diverse and vibrant northern city. Both the university and medical school are large and the city is flooded with students during term time.

The medical school benefits from having the world-renowned specialist cancer hospital The Christie available to students and students who speak a second language can spend time at a European university during their final year.

Course Information

Course Programmes	Standard (A106) Foundation (A104)	**Course Length**	5 years 6 years (Foundation)
Course Type	PBL	**Degree Awarded**	MBChB
Year Size	380	**University Type**	City

Entry Requirements

	Students	Graduates
Typical Offer	AAAb	2:1
Required Subjects	Chemistry and Biology, Maths or Physics	Life science degree
Admission Tests	UKCAT	UKCAT

Admission Statistics

	Standard	Foundation
Applicants	2700	900
Interviews	850	350
Places	380	20
Applicants per Place	8:1	10:1
Open Days	June, Sept, Oct	**International Places** 29

The Interview

Format	MMI
Length	7 station 6 minutes each (42)
When	Dec-March

Course Overview

The five-year programme is made up of three Phases.

Phase 1 (Years 1-2)

Phase 1 is specifically designed to provide you with a firm foundation of knowledge of biomedical, clinical, behavioural and social sciences. There is a focus on practical skills with weekly anatomy dissection classes. Throughout Phase 1 there are regular visits to teaching hospitals and GP practices.

Phase 2 (Years 3-4)

Phase 2 features fully integrated clinical and scientific learning with an increasing emphasis on clinical practice and the acquisition of clinical competence.

Phase 3 (Year 5)

Phase 3 is a transition period where students prepare to become foundation doctors and take on responsibility for patient care. Preparation for practice involves carefully designed work-based assessments.

Hospitals

Manchester Royal Infirmary	2 Minutes	Hope Hospital	20 Minutes
Manchester South	15 Minutes	Royal Preston Hospital	55 Minutes

Insider's Edge

Most freshers stay in halls at Fallowfield which is around ten minutes from the university campus by bus. There is lots to do from watching the Manchester Derby to visiting the Trafford Centre or venturing further afield to the Peak District for a break from city life.

Don't forget your swipe card for the Stopford Building. If you don't have it you won't get in no matter how nicely you ask.

Also, be careful walking up the steps, they are oddly spaced and even have their own Facebook group because of it.

NEWCASTLE

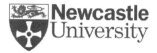

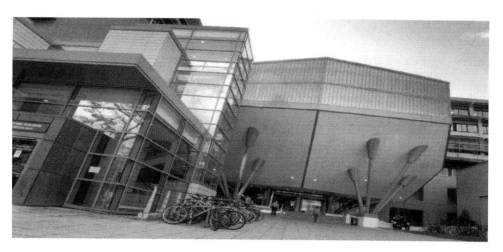

CONTACT DETAILS

Administrator for Admissions
Faculty Undergraduate Office
Medical School
Newcastle University
Newcastle upon Tyne NE2 4HH

t: +44 (0)191 222 7005
e: medic.ugadmin@ncl.ac.uk
http://www.ncl.ac.uk/mbbs/

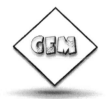

The medical school at Newcastle is a regional medical school and has partnerships with Durham University and the Northern Region NHS. Students are divided between either Newcastle or Durham for the phase 1 (preclinical) years and can choose which campus they would prefer when applying through UCAS.

Clinical placements are spread throughout the Northern region and students train at a variety of clinical bases between Tyneside, Teeside, Wearside and Northumbria.

Newcastle is a fantastic city and Geordies are extremely friendly and obsessed with football.

Course Information

Course Programmes	Standard (A100) GEM (A101)	**Course Length**	5 years 4 years (GEM)
Course Type	Integrated	**Degree Awarded**	MBBS
Year Size	318	**University Type**	City

Entry Requirements

	Students	Graduates
Typical Offer	AAA	2:1
Required Subjects	Chemistry or Biology	Any degree subject
Admission Tests	UKCAT	UKCAT

Admission Statistics

	Standard	GEM
Applicants	2500	1000
Interviews	850	500
Places	318	25
Applicants per Place	7:1	25:1
Open Days	July	**International Places** 22

The Interview

	Students	GEM
Format	Traditional	Traditional
Length	25 Mins	25 Mins
When	Nov-March	Nov-March

Course Overview

Phase I (Years 1 - 2)

You can choose to spend Phase I either at Newcastle University or Durham University, Queen's Campus, Stockton.

Whilst there are certain differences between the course at Newcastle and Durham, the two separate Phase I pathways share common outcomes. The quality of teaching is also excellent at both institutions.

In Phase I your timetable is planned in such a way as to ensure that you spend no more than 50 per cent of your time in scheduled teaching sessions, including the acquisition of early clinical skills. The remainder of your time will be focused on self-directed learning and in gaining early clinical experience.

Phase II (Years 3, 4 and 5)

Regardless of whether you spent Phase I in Newcastle or at Durham University's Queen's Campus in Stockton, all students are integrated into a single common pathway for the three years of Phase II training.

During years 3, 4 and 5 you are allocated to one of four regional Clinical Base Units, which may entail you living away from Newcastle.

In year 4 there is an 18-week period of Student Selected Components and an 8 week Elective.

In the final year, following the final-year examination, you undertake a short preparatory 'shadowing' course to ease your transition from student to your Foundation Programme.

Hospitals

Royal Victoria Infirmary	1 Minute	University Hospital Durham	30 Minutes
Newcastle General Hospital	10 Minutes	Sunderland Royal Hospital	40 Minutes

Insider's Edge

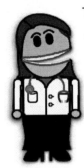

The halls of residence are spread out across the city and students rent from year two onwards. Rent is very reasonable and Newcastle has a relatively low cost of living. The nightlife is incredible with some amazing bars and clubs around the Quayside and city centre.

Make sure you bring warm clothes as Newcastle is on the same latitude as Moscow.

Geordies love Newcastle United and you should try to get to see a match at St James' Park as it is amazing hearing 54,000 fans cheering (or booing) their team.

NORWICH: EAST ANGLIA

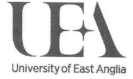

University of East Anglia

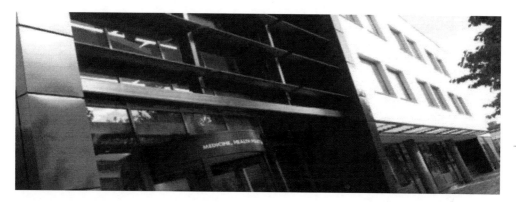

CONTACT DETAILS

University of East Anglia Medical School,
Norwich Research Park,
Norwich, NR4 7TJ

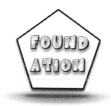

t: +44 (0)1603 591515
e: admissions@uea.ac.uk
http://www.uea.ac.uk/medicine

UEA medical school is relatively new and utilises a modern problem-based learning teaching style. The year group is small making it easy to get to know your peers.

Tho medical school campus Is a ten-minutes walk from the city centre and features modern facilities. The city of Norwich boasts medieval architecture such as the Cathedral and Castle and are a reminder of Norwich's medieval roots as England's second largest city. Norwich offers modern shopping centres and night time venues while surrounded by countryside, allowing students to enjoy themselves in a relaxed environment.

Course Information

Course Programmes	Standard (A100) Foundation (A104)	**Course Length**	5 years 6 years (Foundation)
Course Type	PBL	**Degree Awarded**	MBBS
Year Size	129	**University Type**	City

Entry Requirements

	Students	Graduates
Typical Offer	AAAb	2:1
Required Subjects	Biology and Chemistry or Physics	Life science degree
Admission Tests	UKCAT	UKCAT

Admission Statistics

	Standard		
Applicants	1400		
Interviews	500		
Places	129	**Open Days**	June, July & Sept
Applicants per Place	10:1	**International Places**	13

The Interview

Format	MMI
Length	7 stations, 5 mins (50)
When	Dec-March

Course Overview

Years 1-2

In year one you will study topics including human life, biological and behavioural sciences, and the science behind the musculoskeletal system. During your second year your studies will also cover cardiology, vascular surgery, stroke medicine and respiratory disease.

Year 3

Year three continues the systems-based teaching with hormone regulation, the kidneys, the urological system, the neurological system and the gastrointestinal system. Clinical attachments become more frequent.

Year 4

In year four you will study obstetrics and gynaecology and psychiatry. You will also have the opportunity to take part in a four-week placement as part of an elective.

Year 5

Year five begins with a 'student assistantship'; a nine-week placement split between a medical and surgical specialty. This will cover practical and logistical aspects of becoming a junior doctor, preparing your for FY1.

Intercalation

Students have the opportunity to undertake an intercalated postgraduate (Masters level) degree course after completing year three or year four. Students can take a masters in clinical research (MRes), in clinical education (MClinEd) or in molecular medicine (MSc).

Hospitals

Norfolk and Norwich University Hospital (NNUH)	2 Minutes	Queen Elizabeth Hospital (QEH)	60 Minutes
James Paget University Hospital (JPUH)	50 Minutes	Ipswich Hospital	90 Minutes

Insider's Edge

Norwich halls of residence have been highly rated in student feedback and are very sociable. 'The Square' is the focus of the university campus and features bars, banks, food halls and laundrettes. The 'Sportspark' is one of the largest indoor sports centres in the UK and features a gym and sports facilities for students.

The city of Norwich is beautiful, and a wonderful and safe place to study. The course is varied and full of patient contact from the outset, so the first weeks are extremely exciting. The local hospitals are of high quality and within easy reach, making placement teaching well worthwhile.

NOTTINGHAM

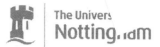

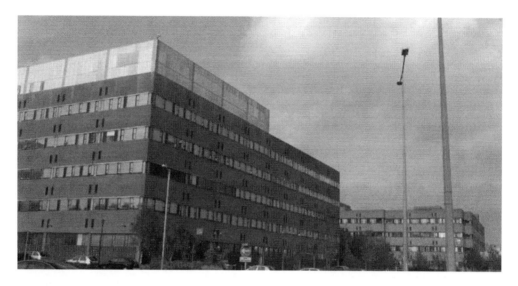

CONTACT DETAILS

Faculty of Medicine and Health Sciences
University of Nottingham
Medical School
Queen's Medical Centre
Nottingham, NG7 2UH

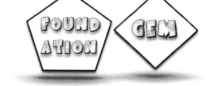

t: +44 (0)115 823 0000
e: medschool@nottingham.ac.uk
http://www.nottingham.ac.uk/mhs/index.aspx

Nottingham medical school opened in 1970 and is centred around one of Britain's busiest teaching hospitals the Queen's Medical Centre. Nottingham students on the standard course are awarded a degree at the end of year 3 (BMedSci) without the need to undertake an additional year of study (the course remains at 5 years).

The university is campus-based with students living at the modern Jubilee campus or the main university campus before moving into rented accommodation in neighbouring Dunkirk or Lenton.

Course Information

Course Programmes	Standard (A100) Foundation (A108) GEM (A101)	**Course Length**	5 years 6 years (Foundation) 4 years (GEM)
Course Type	Integrated	**Degree Awarded**	BMedSci (BMBS for GEM)
Year Size	240	**University Type**	Campus

Entry Requirements

	Students	Graduates
Typical Offer	AAAb	2:1
Required Subjects	Chemistry and Biology	Any degree subject
Admission Tests	UKCAT	GAMSAT

Admission Statistics

	Standard	GEM	Foundation
Applicants	2500	500	350
Interviews	800	200	75
Places	240	90	25
Applicants per Place	10:1	6:1	14:1
Open Days	July	**International Places**	25

The Interview

	Students	GEM/Foundation
Format	MMI	MMI
Length	8 Stations 6 Mins (48)	8 Stations 6 Mins (48)
When	Dec-March	Dec-March

Course Overview

Years 1 - 2

During these two years, core sciences and systems of the body are taught in an integrated manner with lectures, group teaching and short clinical placements.

Year 3

You will undertake an integrated research-based project of your choice and receive a BMedSci at the end of your third year. During this supervised project you will learn to appraise scientific papers and to use research methods.

Years 3-4

During this 17-week phase, students from both standard and GEM courses undertake modules in Clinical Practice (Medicine and Surgery), Community Follow-up and Therapeutics. This period represents the start of intensive clinical teaching and experience.

Year 5

In your final year, you will undertake an elective period when you may experience healthcare abroad. Shadowing courses take place at the end of the final year just before you start working as a new doctor in August.

Four-year (GEM) course structure

The four-year GEM course aims to widen access for a broader range of applicants than school-leavers with A levels. It is intended to build on the intellectual skills acquired by students who have undertaken a first degree. You will be based in a purpose-built medical school building at Royal Derby Hospital for the first 18 months of your course.

After these 18 months, you will then progress onto the clinical phases of the course, joining the students from the undergraduate course and participating in the same attachments at a variety of clinical sites in the East Midlands.

Hospitals

Queens Medical Centre	10 Minutes	Derby Royal Hospital	45 Minutes
Nottingham City Hospital	20 Minutes	Boston Hospital	90 Minutes

Insider's Edge

The campus style of accommodation allows for cheap living and a fantastic student atmosphere with bars and facilities around the campus. Both the students' union and medical society organise lots of events for you to meet other students and there is plenty to do around the city centre.

While Medlink and Medsim are expensive and run by a motivational speaker they do offer insight into life at Nottingham medical school.

OXFORD

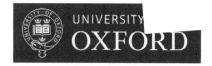

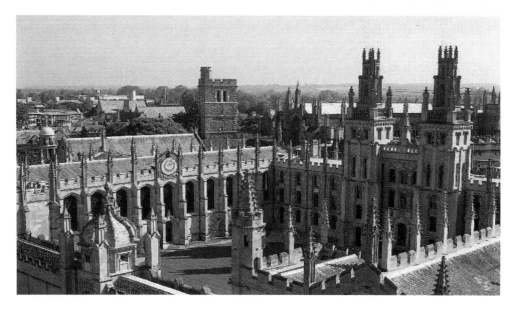

CONTACT DETAILS

Medical Sciences Office,
John Radcliffe Hospital,
Oxford, OX3 9DU

t: +44 (0)1865 270000
e: enquiries@medsci.ox.ac.uk

http://www.medsci.ox.ac.uk/study/medicine/clinical

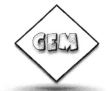

Oxford is the oldest university in the English-speaking world and is known for its 700 year history, academic excellence and tradition. The stunning architecture make Oxford a beautiful place to live and investments, including in the medical students club, Osler House, have provided outstanding facilities in which students can learn, relax, play sport and socialise.

Oxford uses a traditional course structure with sciences taught separately from clinical medicine. In the clinical years you will either stay in Oxford or move to hospitals in London.

Course Information

Course Programmes	Standard (A100) GEM (A101)	**Course Length**	6 years 4 years (GEM)
Course Type	Traditional	**Degree Awarded**	BM BCh
Year Size	150	**University Type**	Collegiate

Entry Requirements

	Students	Graduates
Typical Offer	AAA	2:1
Required Subjects	Chemistry and Biology, Maths or Physics	Life sciences degree
Admission Tests	BMAT	BMAT

Admission Statistics

	Standard	GEM
Applicants	1500	300
Interviews	425	100
Places	150	30
Applicants per Place	10:1	10:1
Open Days	July	**International Places** 14

The Interview

	Students	GEM
Format	Oxbridge	Oxbridge
Length	College Specific	College Specific
When	Dec-March	Dec-March

Course Overview

Preclinical (Years 1-3)

In the first 5 terms there is focus on an introduction to the fundamental aspects of the structure and function of the human body, and to the basis mechanisms underlying disease. Physiology, anatomy and pathology are all taught individually in small groups and lectures. In the remaining 4 terms students undertake a BA in Medical Sciences involving a research project and extended essay.

Clinical (Years 4-6)

After the third year there is competitive entry to the clinical years with students allocated to Oxford or London hospitals depending on their preferences. The core curriculum focus is on preparation for Foundation Training.

Hospitals

John Radcliffe, Oxford	5 Minutes	Banbury	35 Minutes
Churchill, Oxford	5 Minutes	Reading	60 Minutes

Insider's Edge

Freshers live in colleges around Oxford. These allow you to meet students from other courses and live in a friendly environment. Get a cheap bike as you'll use it for everything. The collegiate system means that students are based in a small, friendly environment, while still having access to the facilities and opportunities of the entire university.

The medical school has lots of weird traditions such as the student pantomime (Tingewick) and 'dissection drinks' when medics enjoy a meet and greet with drinks that resemble bodily fluids.

PENINSULA

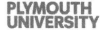

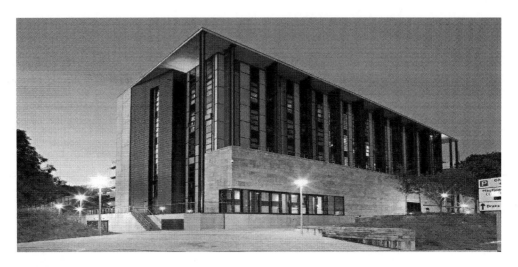

CONTACT DETAILS

Roland Levinsky Building
Plymouth University
Drake Circus
Plymouth
Devon
PL4 8AA

t: +44 (0)1752585858
e: prospectus@plymouth.ac.uk
http://www1.plymouth.ac.uk/peninsula/Pages/default.aspx

Peninsula Medical School offers students a range of settings in which to study from the beaches of Cornwall to the busy streets of Plymouth.

Peninsula is one of the newest medical schools in the UK. Founded in 2002 by Professor John Tooke, the school uses innovative teaching techniques and early clinical exposure to equip students with the knowledge and skills needed to work in the ever-changing world of the modern NHS.

Course Information

Course Programmes	Standard (A100)	**Course Length**	5 years
Course Type	PBL	**Degree Awarded**	BMBS
Year Size	215	**University Type**	City

Entry Requirements

	Students	Graduates
Typical Offer	AAAb	2:1
Required Subjects	Chemistry and Biology or Physics	Life sciences degree
Admission Tests	UKCAT	GAMSAT

Admission Statistics

	Standard		
Applicants	2000		
Interviews	800		
Places	215	**Open Days**	July
Applicants per Place	10:1	**International Places**	16

The Interview

Format	Traditional
Length	20 Minutes
When	Dec-March

COURSE OVERVIEW

Years 1 - 2

Years one and two use problem based learning to teach you about the human life cycle and healthcare provision for both the individual and the wider community.

Years 3 - 4

In years three and four you will rotate through a series of hospital and community placements to gain clinical experience.

Year 5

The emphasis in year five is on the practical implementation of what you've learnt during years one to four and is the final preparation for medical practice. The elective takes place in year five and then students undertake a series of 'apprenticeship attachments' to prepare them for F1.

Hospitals

Truro	2 Minutes	Torbay	10 Minutes
Exeter DGH	5 Minutes	Derriford Hospital	10 Minutes
Royal Devon and Exeter	5 Minutes		

Insider's Edge

Peninsula is in a fantastic location with beaches on your doorstep and the stunning Dartmoor countryside close by.

The medical society organises all the normal social events but also takes advantages of the surroundings with horse-riding in Dartmoor and beach parties in the summer.

Professor Sir John Tooke, the founder of the medical school, led the independent inquiry into 'Modernising Medical Careers', the postgraduate training structure for medical doctors in the UK.

SHEFFIELD

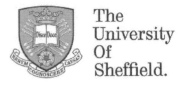

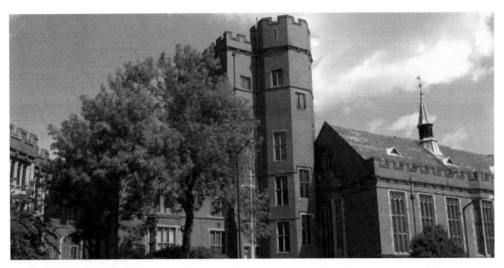

CONTACT DETAILS

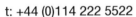

The Medical School
University of Sheffield
Beech Hill Road
Sheffield
S10 2RX

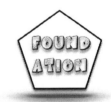

t: +44 (0)114 222 5522
e: medadmissions@sheffield.ac.uk
http://www.shef.ac.uk/medicine

Sheffield is known for its steel and the Snooker World Championship at the Crucible. It is a vibrant and exciting city with the Peak District on its doorstep.

The city, the university and the medical school are a mixture of tradition and new developments, with the Students' Union renowned as one of the liveliest in the United Kingdom.

Sheffield offers an integrated medical course in an organised and friendly environment.

Course Information

Course Programmes	Standard (A100) Foundation (A104)	**Course Length**	5 years 6 years (Foundation)
Course Type	Integrated	**Degree Awarded**	MBChB
Year Size	241	**University Type**	City

Entry Requirements

	Students	Graduates
Typical Offer	AAAb	2:1
Required Subjects	Chemistry and Biology or Physics	Life sciences degree
Admission Tests	UKCAT	UKCAT

Admission Statistics

	Standard		
Applicants	2500		
Interviews	700		
Places	241	**Open Days**	July
Applicants per Place	10:1	**International Places**	18

The Interview

Format	MMI
Length	6 Stations 8 Minutes (48)
When	Jan-March

Course Overview

Phase 1 (Years 1 - 2)

Years one and two teach you about the systems of the body. Phase 1 includes three weeks of Intensive Clinical Experience (ICE), which introduces you to working on the ward with doctors, nurses and other healthcare professionals.

Phase 2 (Years 2 - 3)

In Phase 2 you will spend most of your time in hospital wards, operating theatres and outpatient clinics, learning the skills that you will need to join the medical profession.

Phase 3 (Years 3 - 4)

Phase 3 takes students into both primary and secondary care with an emphasis on clinical medicine.

Phase 4 (Year 5)

From January till June of the final year, you will be immersed in clinical medicine. You will shadow junior doctors to allow you to develop the skills you require to become a Foundation Year 1 doctor.

Hospitals

Royal Hallamshire Hospital	2 Minutes	Bassetlaw hospital	30 Minutes
Northern General Hospital	20 Minutes	Chesterfield Royal Hospital	45 Minutes
Rotherham Hospital	20 Minutes	Pontefract Hospital	50 Minutes
Doncaster Hospital	30 Minutes	Grimsby Hospital	60 Minutes
Barnsley Hospital	30 Minutes	Scunthorpe Hospital	60 Minutes

Insider's Edge

Sheffield is a huge student city. There are loads of bars, clubs and societies offering student nights and activities.

The city itself is modern and clean and the medical school benefits from strong links to surgery via Cutler's Hall and has two large teaching hospitals located within Sheffield.

The Peak District is only 20 minutes away and the city has great transport links with a modern and easily-accessible train station.

SOUTHAMPTON

UNIVERSITY OF
Southampton

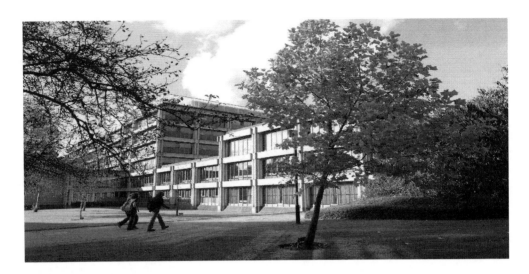

CONTACT DETAILS

Building 85,
Life Sciences Building,
Highfield Campus,
University Rd,
Southampton SO17 1BJ

t: +44 (0)23 8059 5571
e: ugapply.fm@southampton.ac.uk
http://www.southampton.ac.uk/medicine

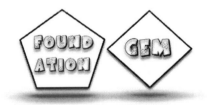

Southampton has a small town feel despite being a large city. The city is one of the greenest in the UK and is bustling with marinas and beautiful heritage attractions. The University is close to the New Forest and historic cities of Winchester and Salisbury and the Isle of Wight is also a short ferry ride away.

The medical school is based at Southampton General Hospital and students are spread across three of the University's six campuses. Students on the standard and foundation courses gain a BMedSc degree on completion of year three in addition to being able to intercalate.

Course Information

Course Programmes	Standard (A100) Foundation (A102) GEM (A101)	**Course Length**	5 years 6 years (Foundation) 4 years (GEM)
Course Type	Integrated	**Degree Awarded**	BM
Year Size	230	**University Type**	City

Entry Requirements

	Students	Graduates
Typical Offer	AAAb	2:1
Required Subjects	Chemistry and Biology	Any Subject
Admission Tests	UKCAT	UKCAT

Admission Statistics

	Standard	Graduate	
Applicants	5000	1200	
Interviews	800	200	
Places	230	40	
Applicants per Place	16:1	30:1	
Open Days	July	**International Places**	24

The Interview

	Students	GEM
Format	Traditional and Group Task	Traditional and Group Task
Length	20 Minutes	20 Minutes
When	Nov-March	Nov-March

Course Overview

Years 1 - 2

In the first two years you will learn about the systems of the body. Within each system, you will integrate your learning of anatomy, biochemistry, pathology, physiology, pharmacology, the social sciences and public health medicine in a clinical context. You will also undertake student selected components in medical humanities, teaching, medical research and a community engagement project.

Year 3

In year three you will undertake a research project followed by clinical placements in hospitals and general practice in the Southampton, Portsmouth and Winchester areas. On successful completion of this year students on the standard five year course will be awarded a Bachelor of Medical Sciences (BMedSc).

Years 4 - 5

In year four you will undertake placements in a range of clinical specialities in Southampton and around the region.

In your final year you will gain experience in a wide range of hospitals, communities and general practices in the south of England and have an opportunity to undertake an elective placement in an area of your choice.

Hospitals

Southampton General	15 Minutes	Salisbury	45 Minutes
Royal South Hants	10 Minutes	Poole	55 Minutes
Winchester	20 Minutes	Frimley Park	1 hour
Portsmouth	30 Minutes	Dorchester	1 hour 20
Basingstoke	40 Minutes	Guildford	1 hour 20
Chichester	45 Minutes	Isle of Wight	1 hour 20
Bournemouth	45 Minutes	Wexham Park, Slough	1 hour 20

Insider's Edge

Southampton medical school offers fantastic support to students and there is always someone to talk to when things are not going well, personally or academically.

The students' union features a club in the basement and Southampton is a vibrant city with plenty of student events arranged through the union and medical society.

Southampton is right on the coast and is ideal for water sports and the Isle of Wight is just a short ferry ride away.

WARWICK

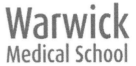

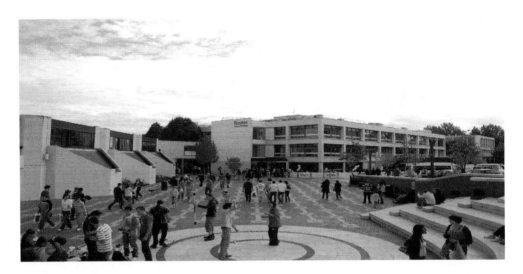

CONTACT DETAILS

Warwick Medical School
The University of Warwick
Coventry
CV4 7AL

t: +44 (0)24 7652 4585

e: wmsinfo@warwick.ac.uk

http://www2.warwick.ac.uk/fac/med/study/ugr/

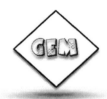

Warwick medical school is located south of Coventry on the border of Warwickshire. Warwick only accepts applications from graduates making the course more mature with emphasis on the needs of the graduate learner.

Graduates from any discipline are welcomed and the campus style of university offers cheap accommodation in a central location.

Built in 2000 the medical school features modern facilities and students also benefit from the teaching facilities at University Hospital in Coventry when on clinical attachments.

Course Information

Course Programmes	GEM (A101) only	**Course Length**	4 years (GEM)
Course Type	Integrated	**Degree Awarded**	MBChB
Year Size	164	**University Type**	Campus

Entry Requirements

	Graduates
Typical Offer	2:1
Required Subjects	Any degree subject
Admission Tests	UKCAT

Admission Statistics

	GEM		
Applicants	1100		
Interviews	350		
Places	164	**Open Days**	Feb, June, Sept
Applicants per Place	6:1	**International Places**	13

The Interview

	Graduates
Format	Selection Centre (Shared with Bart's)
Length	Half-Day
When	Feb

Course Overview

Years 1-2

Year one features integrated teaching, including clinical exposure in hospital settings. You will be allocated to small learning groups made up of around ten students.

In year two more focus is placed on clinical teaching in both hospital and community settings.

Years 3-4

The majority of your learning will be based in the community and in hospitals through partner trusts and centred around three specialist clinical placements.

Year four builds on year three with two further specialist clinical placements. The elective period also takes place in year four as students prepare for working as foundation doctors.

Hospitals

University Hospital	15 Minutes	George Eliot Hospital	30 Minutes
Warwick Hospital	20 Minutes	Alexandra Hospital	40 Minutes

Insider's Edge

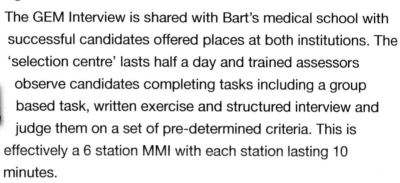

The GEM Interview is shared with Bart's medical school with successful candidates offered places at both institutions. The 'selection centre' lasts half a day and trained assessors observe candidates completing tasks including a group based task, written exercise and structured interview and judge them on a set of pre-determined criteria. This is effectively a 6 station MMI with each station lasting 10 minutes.

Phase I can be pretty tough, they don't call it "fast-track" and "intensive" for nothing. You spend most days working from 9am to 5pm. As an entirely postgraduate course most people have spent years getting here and there is a real sense of family and camaraderie.

The central campus offers lots of sports and leisure facilities, which are available to students. Even though it is a graduate-only course the medical society still organises lots of fun social events to help you relax and enjoy your time at Warwick.

Wales

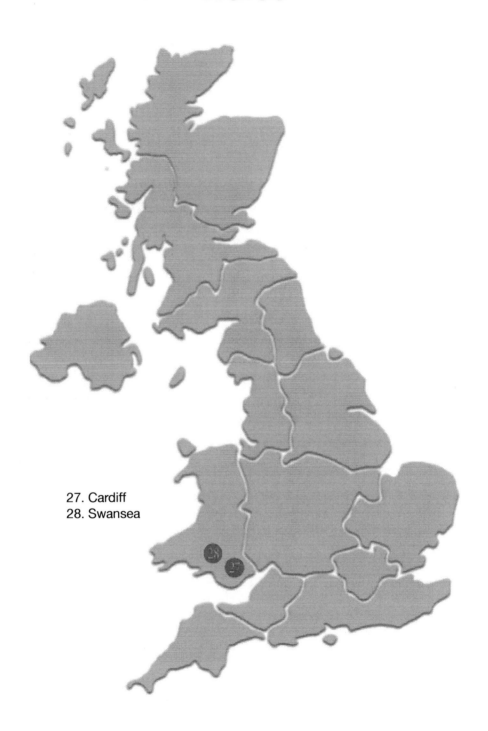

27. Cardiff
28. Swansea

CARDIFF

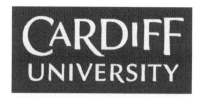

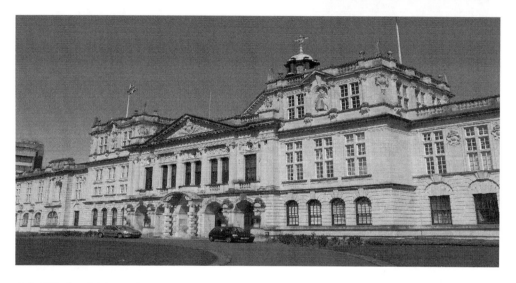

CONTACT DETAILS

Cardiff University School of Medicine
Cochrane Medical Education Centre
Heath Park
Cardiff CF14 4YU

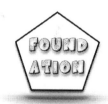

t: +44 (0)29 20 68 8113
e: medadmissions@cardiff.ac.uk
http://medicine.cf.ac.uk

Cardiff medical school is the only undergraduate medical school in Wales. Cardiff is a modern and vibrant city and the city centre is flooded with students during term time.

The medical school is large and offers an integrated course. Students may be sent as far as Bangor for clinical attachments and benefit from the large University Hospital of Wales and it's teaching facilities.

Course Information

Course Programmes	Standard (A100) Foundation (A108)	Course Length	5 years 6 years (Foundation)
Course Type	Integrated	Degree Awarded	MBChB
Year Size	300	University Type	City

Entry Requirements

	Students	Graduates
Typical Offer	AAAb	2:1
Required Subjects	Two from: Chemistry, Biology, Maths and Physics	Life sciences degree
Admission Tests	UKCAT	UKCAT

Admission Statistics

	Standard		
Applicants	3000		
Interviews	850		
Places	300	Open Days	June & July
Applicants per Place	10:1	International Places	28

The Interview

Format	Traditional
Length	20 Minutes
When	Nov-March

Course Overview

Years 1 - 2

Your first two years are integrated and you will be learning core science and clinical practice simultaneously with early clinical attachments.

Years 3 - 4

During years three and four you will spend most of your time on clinical placements as you learn medicine by following patients through the healthcare system.

In year three you will have opportunities for multiple short projects or a single longitudinal study, while in year four a 'Science in Practice' block will give you exposure to leading University and NHS experts and researchers.

Year 5

Year five features the 'Harmonisation Programme' or senior student assistantship, allowing you to work as part of a clinical team. This will take place in the hospital where you will undertake your first Foundation (F1) job, if it is in Wales, to prepare you for life after graduation.

Placements will be followed by an 8-10 week student elective at a destination of your choice, anywhere in the world.

Hospitals

University Hospital of Wales	3 Minutes	Singleton Hospital, Swansea	1 Hour
Llandough Hospital	20 Minutes	Morriston Hospital, Swansea	1 Hour
Royal Gwent, Newport	20 Minutes	West Wales General Hospital, Carmarthen	1 Hour 20 Minutes
Royal Glamorgan Hospital, Llantrisant	25 Minutes	Withybush General Hospital, Haverfordwest	1 Hour 40 Minutes
Princess of Wales, Bridgend	25 Minutes	Brongalis General Hospital, Aberystwyth	2 Hours 30 Minutes
Prince Charles, Merthyr Tydfil	40 Minutes	Wrexham Maelor Hospital, Wrexham	3 Hours
Neath Port Talbot Hospital, Port Talbot	50 Minutes	Glan Clwyd Hospital, Rhyl	3 Hours 40 Minutes
Neville Hall Hospital, Abergavenny	55 Minutes	Ysbyty Gwynedd, Bangor	4 Hours 20 Minutes

Insider's Edge

Freshers live in halls located around the city. From year two onwards students rent in areas such as Cathays around the main campus and rent is relatively cheap for a major city.

Cardiff medics have their own bar which gives students a place to be during their lunch breaks and is sometimes used in the evenings for socials. The main student union has its own club and bar with regular live bands and Cardiff nightlife is safe and exciting.

Visiting the Millennium Stadium is a necessity with cheap tickets for the smaller games and a fantastic atmosphere during the Six Nations matches.

SWANSEA

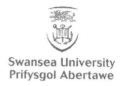

Swansea University
Prifysgol Abertawe

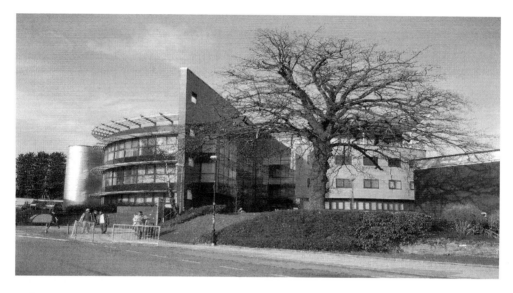

CONTACT DETAILS

College of Medicine
Grove Building
Swansea University
Singleton Park
Swansea
SA2 8PP

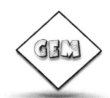

t: +44 (0)1792 513400
e: medicine@swansea.ac.uk
http://www.swansea.ac.uk/medicine

Established in 2004 Swansea medical school offers a small, graduate-only course with the four-year course designed specifically for the needs of graduate medics.

Graduates from any discipline are welcomed and will need to sit the GAMSAT admission test before applying. The seaside city of Swansea features natural beauty with the Gower Peninsula and Rhosilli Bay just minutes away.

Course Information

Course Programmes	GEM (A101) only	Course Length	4 years (GEM)
Course Type	Integrated	Degree Awarded	MBChB
Year Size	70	University Type	City

Entry Requirements

	Graduates
Typical Offer	2:1
Required Subjects	Any degree subject
Admission Tests	GAMSAT

Admission Statistics

	GEM		
Applicants	700		
Interviews	160		
Places	70	Open Days	March & June
Applicants per Place	10:1	International Places	0

The Interview

	Graduates
Format	Selection Centre
Length	Two 20 Minute Traditional Interviews and 30 Minute Written Task
When	Feb

Course Overview

The programme consists of two phases.

Phase 1

Teaching is organised into 'Learning Weeks' featuring case-based discussions. You will participate in Community-Based Learning (CBL) in General Practice for one day every third week and Learning Opportunities in the Clinical Setting (LOCS) from early on in the course. Phase I tends to have more of a preclinical focus while integrating exposure to clinical experience.

Phase 2

Phase two features more exposure to clinical practice and community based learning. The elective takes place at the end of year three and is a six-week clinical placement that may be taken overseas.

There is a shadowing period at end of year four before beginning Foundation jobs.

Hospitals

Singleton General Hospital	On site	Cefn Coed Psychiatric Hospital	20 Minutes
Morriston Infirmary	20 Minutes		

Insider's Edge

Most students choose to live in the Hendrefoilan Student Village, a residential area for students. Rented accommodation is also very affordable.The university has plenty of sports and leisure facilities with cheap rates for students.

There is no better place to relax and unwind than on the sandy beaches or the Gower Peninsula. For more active students there are plenty of water sports available including surfing and kite-surfing.

Scotland

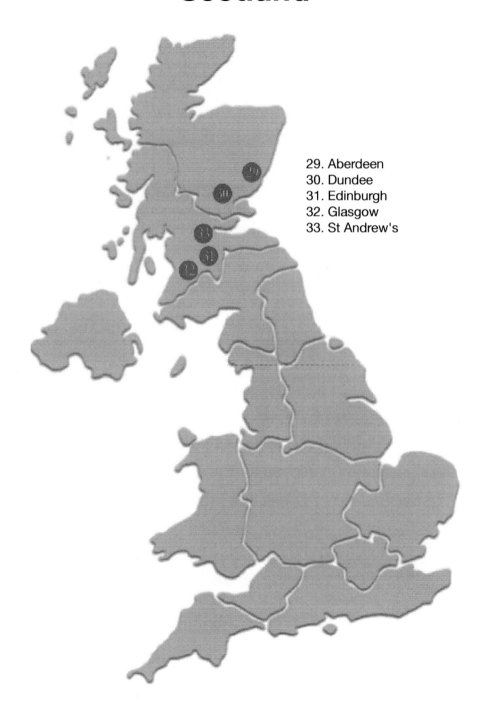

29. Aberdeen
30. Dundee
31. Edinburgh
32. Glasgow
33. St Andrew's

ABERDEEN

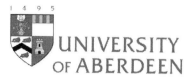

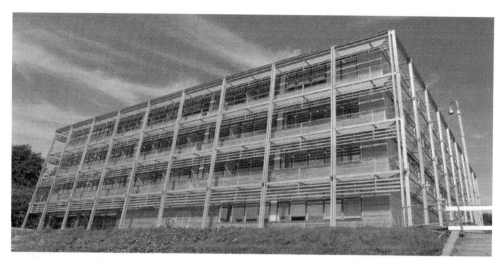

CONTACT DETAILS

Aberdeen School of Medicine and Dentistry
3rd Floor,
Polwarth Building,
Foresterhill,
Aberdeen,
AB25 2ZD

http://www.abdn.ac.uk/medicine/prospective/

The University of Aberdeen was founded in 1495, making it the UK's fifth oldest University. It is a small but beautifully preserved university

The medical school is over 500 years old and is located in the Foresterhill campus approximately two miles from the centre of Aberdeen.

The Suttie Centre, a purpose-built teaching centre for healthcare professionals, offers modern teaching facilities and modern learning tools such as a simulated ward area. The 'Remote and Rural' placement offers students in the clinical years an opportunity to experience medicine in the remote locations off the Scottish coast such as Orkney and the Shetlands.

Course Information

Course Programmes	Standard (A100)	Course Length	5 years
Course Type	Integrated	Degree Awarded	MBChB
Year Size	168	University Type	City

Entry Requirements

	Students	Graduates
Typical Offer	AAA	2:1
Required Subjects	Chemistry and Biology, Maths or Physics	Life sciences degree
Admission Tests	UKCAT	UKCAT

Admission Statistics

	Standard		
Applicants	1500		
Interviews	700		
Places	168	Open Days	August & Sept
Applicants per Place	10:1	International Places	16

The Interview

Format	MMI
Length	7 Stations, 7 Mins (49)
When	Nov-March

Course Overview

Years 1-2

The first year starts by providing you with the knowledge and understanding of medical sciences and disease.

In year two systems-based teaching and the Community Course develop your knowledge and skills. Two four-week SSC periods will allow you to study a topic in more detail.

Years 3-4

The study of the systems and the Community Course is completed in year three. The SSC in third year provides a unique opportunity to study Medical Humanities for a six week module. You will get to experience a wide range of biweekly clinical attachments and, by the end of the year, you will be able to perform a complete head-to-toe examination of a patient.

In year four students undertake nine five-week clinical blocks in many different clinical areas and disciplines.

Year 5

Year five is an apprentice year where students prepare for professional practice as a doctor. Some students may wish to continue to undertake Remote and Rural attachments for a second year for some or all of year five.

Hospital

Royal Cornhill Hospital	5 Minutes	Woodend	15 Minutes
Foresterhill	7 Minutes		

Insider's Edge

The admissions procedure at Aberdeen gives weighting to different aspects of your application including academic predictions (25%), UKCAT (8%), the UCAS written application (22%) then subsequent interview performance (45%).

Aberdeen is a costal city with everything within walking distance. There are plenty of vibrant bars and The Lemon Tree is a popular venue attracting live bands and comedy.

The medical society also organise plenty of events and the Freshers' Fling is a great way to meet people and is an unforgettable evening.

DUNDEE

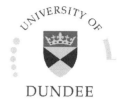

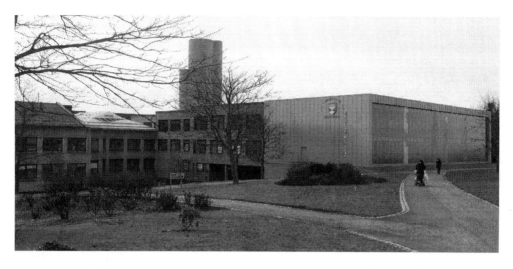

CONTACT DETAILS

Ninewells Hospital & Medical School
Dundee
Scotland, UK
DD1 9SY

t: +44 (0)1382 384697

e: asrs-medicine@dundee.ac.uk

http://modicino.dundoo.ac.uk

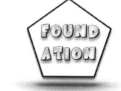

Dundee medical school offers a fully integrated course with extensive teaching and research facilities.

Ninewells Hospital and medical school is the centre of many areas of forefront and pioneering research in areas including cancer, diabetes, cardiovascular disease, drug development, and medical education.

The modern Dow clinical simulation suite provides students with opportunities for clinical skills teaching. Dundee itself is a friendly, coastal Scottish city with plenty for students to do.

Course Information

Course Programmes	Standard (A100) Foundation (A104)	**Course Length**	5 years 6 years (Foundation)
Course Type	Integrated	**Degree Awarded**	MBChB
Year Size	340	**University Type**	City

Entry Requirements

	Students	Graduates
Typical Offer	AAA	2:1
Required Subjects	Chemistry and Biology or Physics	Life sciences degree
Admission Tests	UKCAT	UKCAT

Admission Statistics

	Standard		
Applicants	1400		
Interviews	550		
Places	134	**Open Days**	July
Applicants per Place	10:1	**International Places**	12

The Interview

Format	MMI
Length	10 Stations, 7 Mins (90)
When	January

Course Overview

Phase 1 (Year 1)

Phase 1 deals with the basic sciences behind medicine. There is early patient contact in the Doctors, Patients and Communities and Clinical Skills programmes.

Phase 2 (Years 2-3)

Semester two of year one and semesters three to six of years two and three form Phase two. Phase two is an integrated body-system-based course that expands the students' understanding from Phase one.

Transition Block

Between years three and four there is a transition period designed to prepare students for the task-based clinical approach adopted in Phase 3.

Phase 3 (Years 4-5)

Years four and five form Phase 3, consisting mainly of clinical attachment blocks. There is a large project similar to a SSC available to complete in year four. The majority of year five is devoted to clinical SSCs together with two foundation apprenticeship attachments.

Hospitals

Ninewells Hospital	15 minutes	Queen Margaret	60 minutes
Perth Royal Infirmary	30 minutes	Airdrie	90 minutes
Kirkcaldy Hospital	45 minutes		

Insider's Edge

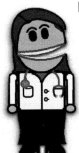

Freshers usually live in halls in the Student Village, located near the main university campus. From year two onwards rent is affordable.

Dundee has a strong association with medical education with many teaching tools developed at the Centre for Medical Education.

Dundee itself is a small city with a large student population and has major transport links to the larger Scottish cities.

Dundee provide a video for those unsure of what the MMI interview format which can be accessed through their admissions website.

EDINBURGH

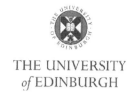

THE UNIVERSITY
of EDINBURGH

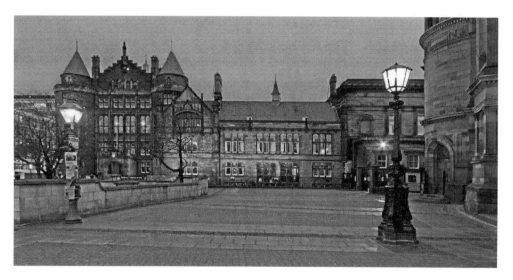

CONTACT DETAILS

College of Medicine The University of Edinburgh
The Queen's Medical Research Institute
47 Little France Crescent
Edinburgh EH16 4TJ

t: +44 (0)131 242 9300
e: mvm@ed.ac.uk
http://www.ed.ac.uk/schools-departments/medicine-vet-medicine/

Located in the Scottish capital, Edinburgh medical school boasts an integrated style of teaching with an excellent anatomy department and links to the Royal College of Surgeons of Edinburgh.

The city of Edinburgh is a vibrant city that is filled with history and beautiful architecture such as Edinburgh castle.

The medical school do not interview school leavers and students benefit from major hospitals such as the Royal Infirmary of Edinburgh and the Royal Hospital for the Sick Children together with useful online facilities.

141

Course Information

Course Programmes	Standard (A100)	Course Length	5 years
Course Type	Integrated	Degree Awarded	MBChB
Year Size	205	University Type	City

Entry Requirements

	Students	Graduates
Typical Offer	AAA	2:1
Required Subjects	Chemistry and Biology, Maths or Physics	Life sciences degree
Admission Tests	UKCAT	UKCAT

Admission Statistics

	Standard		
Applicants	2000		
Interviews	700		
Places	205	Open Days	June & Sept
Applicants per Place	10:1	International Places	15

The Interview

	Students	Graduates (For standard course)
Format		MMI
Length	Edinburgh do not routinely interview school leavers	3 Stations, 10 Mins (30)
When		Nov-March

Course Overview

Years 1 - 2

You will study the biomedical and clinical sciences such as anatomy, physiology, pharmacology, pathology and microbiology of a system along with relevant social and ethical aspects of clinical practice.

Practical, clinical and research skills are developed through workshops, community projects, GP-based teaching and three student selected components or projects on a range of topics from the clinical to the non-medical.

Years 3 - 4

Modules take you through the major systems-based clinical specialities, in hospital and community-attachments.

Year 5

In year five you will learn in an apprenticeship model to prepare for the F1 year. Students also undertake an eight-week elective period.

Hospitals

Royal Infirmary of Edinburgh	0 Minutes	Queen Margaret Hospital, Dunfermline	50 Minutes
Royal Hospital for the Sick Children	15 Minutes	Falkirk Hospital	60 Minutes
Western General	30 Minutes	Kirkcaldy	60 Minutes
Borders General Hospital	45 Minutes	Dumfries & Galloway	90 Minutes
Haddington/ Roodlands	45 Minutes		

Insider's Edge

The majority of Freshers live in halls of residence such as Pollock Halls or one of the many self-catering options spread throughout the city. Rent from year two onwards is fairly expensive, though this can be minimised by moving in with three-four other students.

There is plenty to do in Edinburgh from visiting Arthur's Seat (an extinct volcano) to watching a rugby game or attending the Fringe festival. The city itself is beautiful and compact with great transport links including a new tram system and a cheap bus to and from the airport.

GLASGOW

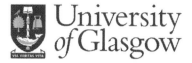

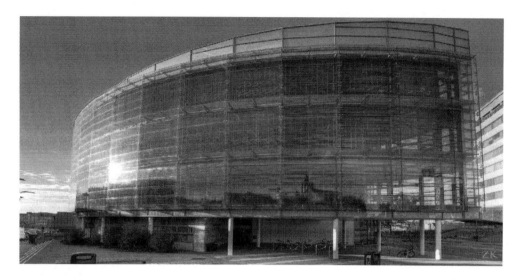

CONTACT DETAILS

Medical School Office
University of Glasgow
Glasgow G12 8QQ

t: +44 (0)141 330 6216

e: med-sch-admissions@glasgow.ac.uk

http://www.gla.ac.uk/schools/medicine/mus/

Glasgow Medical School is located in the Wolfson Building. Teaching methods include problem based learning scenarios and clinical skills training. These are taught in a purpose-built clinical skills suite, which contains its own mock hospital ward and consultation rooms.

The university itself was founded in 1451 and offers plenty of facilities for students.

Course Information

Course Programmes	Standard (A100)	Course Length	5 years
Course Type	PBL	Degree Awarded	MBChB
Year Size	230	University Type	City

Entry Requirements

	Students	Graduates
Typical Offer	AAA	2:1
Required Subjects	Chemistry and Biology, Maths or Physics	Life sciences degree
Admission Tests	UKCAT	UKCAT

Admission Statistics

	Standard		
Applicants	2000		
Interviews	700		
Places	230	Open Days	June, Sept, Oct
Applicants per Place	9:1	International Places	18

The Interview

Format	Traditional
Length	20 Minutes
When	Nov-March

Course Overview

Phase 1

During Phase 1 you will be taught the fundamentals of biomedical science, and the skills necessary for self-directed learning. The themes covered in this section include homeostasis, basic anatomy, physiology and biochemistry, and the fundamentals of health and illness in communities.

Phase 2

Phase 2 takes up the second half of first year and all of year two. This is a system-based, integrated approach to biomedical sciences and basic clinical problems relating to individual systems.

Phase 3

Phase 3 takes up the first 15 weeks of third year, during which time you will move from the University campus and spend more time in the teaching hospitals in Glasgow and in the wider West of Scotland. Through regular clinical bedside teaching you will develop clinical skills in the hospital and general practice environment.

During the summer vacations after third and fourth years you will be required to undertake two four-week periods of elective study.

Phase 4

Phase 4 comprises of the second half of year 3, all of year 4 and year 5 up to graduation. This is the final part of the programme, during which you will be attached to clinical specialties, including obstetrics and gynaecology, child health, psychological medicine, general practice, and more specialised aspects of medicine and surgery. During this phase you will spend most of your time in hospital attachments in Glasgow and in the wider west of Scotland and learn the clinical and practical skills necessary to work as a junior doctor.

Hospitals

Western Infirmary	2 Minutes	Royal Alexandria Hospital, Paisley	40 Minutes
Gartnavel General and Gartnavel Royal (Psychiatric Hospital)	10 Minutes	Hairmyres Hospital	45 Minutes
Glasgow Royal Infirmary	15 Minutes	Wilshaw Hospital	45 Minutes
The Royal Hospital for Sick Children, Yorkhill	15 Minutes	Crosshouse Hospital	60 Minutes
Southern General	20 Minutes	Ayr Hospital	90 Minutes

Insider's Edge

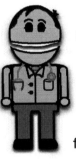

Students tend to live in halls of residence or in the city's West End. Rent is fairly cheap for a major city as is cost of living and transport.

Glasgow has two students' unions and there are a number of fun societies to join once you arrive.

ST ANDREWS

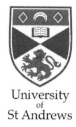

University
of
St Andrews

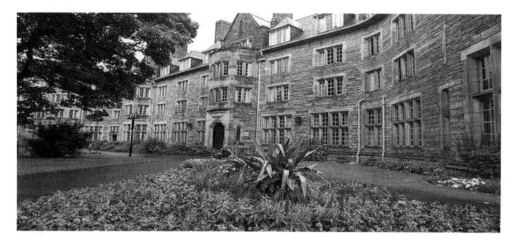

CONTACT DETAILS

School of Medicine
University of St Andrews
Medical and Biological Sciences Building
North Haugh
St Andrews
KY16 9TF

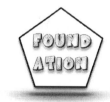

t: +44 (0)1334 461851

e: medicine@st-and.ac.uk

http://medicine.st-andrews.ac.uk

Medicine has been taught in the historic Scottish town of St Andrews since 1413.

St Andrews provides teaching for the preclinical years only with students moving on to a partnered medical school for their clinical training. There is a strong focus on clinical sciences and the small year size makes teaching personal and friendly.

Course Information

Course Programmes	Standard (A100) (clinical years at partnered medical schools)	**Course Length**	3 years (out of 6)
Course Type	Traditional	**Degree Awarded**	BSc (MBChB at partnered university)
Year Size	160	**University Type**	City

Entry Requirements

	Students	Graduates
Typical Offer	AAA	2:1
Required Subjects	Chemistry and Biology, Maths or Physics	Life sciences degree
Admission Tests	UKCAT	UKCAT

Admission Statistics

	Standard		
Applicants	1600		
Interviews	400		
Places	160	**Open Days**	Yearlong
Applicants per Place	10:1	**International Places**	30

The Interview

Format	MMI
Length	4 Stations 7 Minutes (28)
When	Nov-March

Course Overview

Students attain a BSc (Hons) in Medicine lasting three years at St Andrews and then undertake the MB ChB, a further three years, at a partnered medical school (Aberdeen, Dundee, Edinburgh, Glasgow or Manchester).

Year 1

Year one covers the clinical sciences including pathology, microbiology, health psychology, public health medicine and key aspects of medical ethics and law. You will discover the basics of medicine on an individual and population level.

Years 2 and 3

The Honours programme comprises a series of modules that revisit and build upon the knowledge base that was established in year one. Body systems will be studied in depth and you will examine the scientific basis of disease and treatments.

Insider's Edge

St Andrew's is a university town with almost everyone you meet having some connection to the University. This makes for a friendly atmosphere and the beautiful architecture and surroundings make for a relaxing place to study.

Despite its small size the numerous student societies provide plenty of fun things to do and there are excellent transport links to the larger Scottish cities.

Northern Ireland

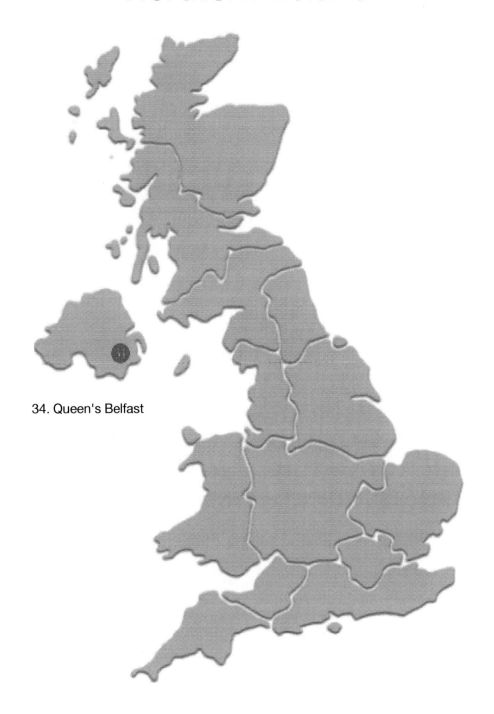

34. Queen's Belfast

Queen's Belfast

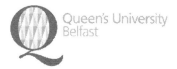

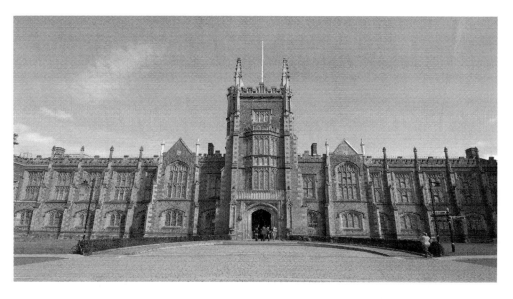

CONTACT DETAILS

Centre for Medical Education
Whitla Medical Building
97 Lisburn Road
Belfast
BT9 7BL

t: +44 (0)2890 972450
e: medicaled@qub.ac.uk

http://www.qub.ac.uk/schools/mdbs/medicine/

Queen's University was founded as a college in 1885, becoming a university in 1909 in the vibrant and student-friendly city of Belfast.

Belfast is a compact city with a dedicated student area giving it a campus-feel with the added benefits of city life. The medical school is based at the Medical Biology Centre (MBC) located in the main university campus, fifteen minutes from the city centre.

Course Information

Course Programmes	Standard (A100)	**Course Length**	5 years
Course Type	Integrated	**Degree Awarded**	MB BCh BAO
Year Size	260	**University Type**	City

Entry Requirements

	Students	Graduates
Typical Offer	AAAb	2:1
Required Subjects	Chemistry and Biology, Maths or Physics	Life sciences degree
Admission Tests	UKCAT	UKCAT

Admission Statistics

	Standard		
Applicants	1400		
Interviews	500		
Places	260	**Open Days**	Feb & Sept
Applicants per Place	5:1	**International Places**	29

The Interview

Format	MMI
Length	9 Stations, 8 Mins (90)
When	Jan-March

Course Overview

At the end of the five year course you receive the degrees of MB BCh BAO.

MB is Bachelor of Medicine

BCh is Bachelor of Surgery

BAO is Bachelor in the Art of Obstetrics

Years 1 - 2

During the first two years of the course you learn about the scientific basis of medicine. You study body systems and pathology, microbiology, therapeutics and genetics. Teaching of basic science subjects is integrated with clinical skills training through clinical simulation and practice with patients.

Year 3

The third year has greater clinical focus. Clinical teaching in each of the medical and surgical disciplines is integrated with therapeutic, pathological and microbiological principles relevant to clinical practice.

Year 4 - 5

During the fourth and fifth years you gain experience in emergency medicine and general practice. In fifth year you undertake an apprenticeship during which you complete work alongside a Foundation Doctor.

Teaching in ethics, communication, teamwork, and related behavioural science is embedded throughout the curriculum.

Hospitals

Royal Victoria Hospital	5 Mins	Craigavon Area Hospital	30 Mins
City Hospital	2 Mins	Altnagelvin Hospital	1hr 15 Mins
Mater Infirmorum Hospital	10 Mins	Causeway Hospital	1hr 30 Mins
Musgrave Park Hospital	10 Mins	Erne Hospital	1hr 30 Mins
Ulster Hospital	20 Mins	Tyrone County	2hrs
Antrim Area Hospital	20 Mins		

Insider's Edge

Queens is the only UK medical school that gives you a BAO (Bachelor of Obstetrics) as well as your normal medical degree.

Freshers tend to live in The Elms halls, a short, twenty-minute walk from the Medical Biology Centre. Rent is reasonable and most students tend to rent in the main student areas each around twenty minutes from the city centre.

There are plenty of student-friendly pubs, bars and societies to keep you occupied and Belfast airport offers cheap flights to England and Europe.

Download The FREE Get Me Into Medical School App Now

We hope you found the book useful and wish you luck in your medical school application.

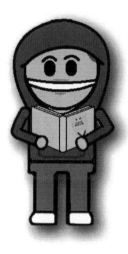

For the latest information be sure to check out featuring free resources

www.getmeintomedicalschool.com

Follow us on Twitter

www.twitter.com/getmeintomed

Like us on Facebook

www.facebook.com/getmeintomedicalschool

13978926R00089

Printed in Great Britain
by Amazon.co.uk, Ltd.,
Marston Gate.